SUICIDE
and the Elderly

RECENT TITLES IN
BIBLIOGRAPHIES AND INDEXES IN GERONTOLOGY

Elder Neglect and Abuse: An Annotated Bibliography
Tanya F. Johnson, James G. O'Brien, and Margaret F. Hudson, compilers

Retirement: An Annotated Bibliography
John J. Miletich, compiler

SUICIDE
and the Elderly

An Annotated Bibliography and Review

Compiled by
Nancy J. Osgood
and John L. McIntosh

Bibliographies and Indexes in Gerontology, Number 3

GREENWOOD PRESS
New York • Westport, Connecticut • London

LIBRARY OF CONGRESS CATALOGING-IN-PUBLICATION DATA

Osgood, Nancy J.
  Suicide and the elderly.

  (Bibliographies and indexes in gerontology,
ISSN 0743-7560 ; no. 3)
  Includes indexes.
  1. Aged—Suicidal behavior—Bibliography.
I. McIntosh, John L. II. Title. III. Series.
Z7164.04083 1986 [HV6546]   016.3622   86-14935
ISBN 0-313-24786-2 (lib. bdg. : alk. paper)

Library of Congress Catalog Card Number: 86-14935
ISBN: 0-313-24786-2
ISSN: 0743-7560

First published in 1986

Greenwood Press, Inc.
88 Post Road West, Westport, Connecticut 06881

Printed in the United States of America

The paper used in this book complies with the
Permanent Paper Standard issued by the National
Information Standards Organization (Z39.48-1984).

10 9 8 7 6 5 4 3 2 1

COPYRIGHT ACKNOWLEDGMENT

Figures 1-5 appear in J. L. McIntosh, "Components of the decline in elderly
suicide: Suicide among the young-old and old-old by race and sex,"
Death Education 8 (1984, Supplement): 113-24. Copyright 1984 by Hemisphere Corporation.

CONTENTS

SERIES FOREWORD

The annotated bibliographies in this series provide answers to the fundamental question, "What is known?" Their purpose is simple, yet profound: to provide comprehensive reviews and references for the work done in various fields of gerontology. They are based on the fact that it is no longer possible for anyone to comprehend the vast body of research and writing in even one sub-specialty without years of work.

This fact has become true only in recent years. When I was an undergraduate (Class of '52) I think no one at Duke had even heard of gerontology. Almost no one in the world was identified as a gerontologist. Now there are over 5,000 professional members of the Gerontological Society of America. There were no courses in gerontology. Now there are thousands of courses offered by most major (and many minor) colleges and universities. There was only one journal (the Journal of Gerontology), begun in 1945. Now there are a dozen professional journals and several dozen books in gerontology published each year.

The reasons for this dramatic growth are well known: the dramatic increase in numbers of aged, the shift from family to public responsibility for the security and care of the elderly, the recognition of aging as a "social problem," and the growth of science in general. It is less well known that this explosive growth in knowledge has developed the need for new solutions to the old problem of comprehending and "keeping up" with a field of knowledge. The old indexes and library card catalogues have become increasingly inadequate for the job. On-line computer indexes and abstracts are one solution, but they make no evaluative selections and do not organize sources logically as is done here.

These bibliographies will be obviously useful for researchers who need to know what research has (or has not) been done in their field. The annotations contain enough information so that the researcher usually does not have to search out the original articles. In the past, the "review of the literature" has often been haphazard and was rarely comprehensive, because of the large investment of time (and money) that would be required by a truly comprehensive review. Now, using these bibliographies, researchers can be more confident that they are not missing important previous research; they can be more confident that they are not duplicating past efforts and "reinventing the wheel." It may well become standard and expected practice for researchers to consult such bibliographies, even before they start their research.

These bibliographies will also be useful reference tools for teachers, students, policy analysts, lawyers, legislators, administrators, and any intelligent person who wishes to find out what is known about a given topic in gerontology.

Suicide among the elderly is an interesting and important topic within Gerontology for several reasons. First, there are the puzzling demographic facts that require explanation. Why do suicides increase among men in old age, but not among women? Why has suicide declined among the elderly, but not among younger people? Then there are the questions of motivation: why do the elderly commit suicide? There are also questions about what could be done to prevent suicides. Finally, there are ethical questions about whether suicide is ever "rational" and desirable.

The authors of this bibliography have done an outstanding job of covering all the relevant information and organizing it into easily accessible form. Not only are there 226 annotated references (with unusually detailed annotations) but there is a comprehensive review of the literature, a list of bibliographic sources on elderly suicide, and a set of demographic tables and figures in the appendix giving detailed statistics on the subject. Thus, one can look for relevant material in this volume in several ways: (1) look up a given subject in the subject index; or (2) look up a given author in the author index; (3) turn to the section in the review of the literature (Chapter 1) that covers the topic; (4) look over the references in Chapters 3, 4, or 5, depending on whether you are interested in overviews and other non-empirical works, empirical investigations, or non-English language works; or (5) use the tables in the appendix for demographic statistics.

The authors of this bibliography are unusually qualified experts in this area because both of them have done previous reviews of suicide among the elderly. Dr. Osgood has written several articles and a book on the topic, and Dr. McIntosh has written several articles and bibliographies.

We believe you will find this volume to be the most useful, comprehensive, and easily accessible reference work in its field. I will appreciate any comments you care to send me.

Erdman B. Palmore
Center for the Study of Aging and Human Development
Duke University Medical Center
Durham, NC 27710

INTRODUCTION

SIGNIFICANCE, GOAL, AND ORGANIZATION

Much has been written recently about suicide, and most of this attention has been focused on young people. The old, however, have 50 percent higher suicide rates than do the young and represent the highest risk age group for suicide. While there have been dozens of books published on youth suicide in recent years, only two have appeared on elderly suicide. They are Marv Miller's (1979, reference 3-027) Suicide After Sixty and Nancy Osgood's (1985, reference 3-034) Suicide in the Elderly. Similarly, much research has been done regarding suicide at young ages but much less has been conducted with respect to the old. The goal of this book is to bring together in one source the accumulated knowledge/reference materials regarding elderly suicide, particularly the research findings. To this end, the book includes a brief review of the literature on elderly suicide, including statistics, theory, assessment, prevention, ethics, and future research needs. The reader is then directed to 450 sources in which future and existing materials on elderly suicide and suicide in general may be found (i.e., bibliographies and index/abstract sources). The largest portion of the book is comprised of annotations of the published (or otherwise available) references on suicide and the elderly, both the empirical investigations as well as non-empirical and overview works. Non-English language works are listed and some are annotated as well. Finally, from the many official statistical sources for the United States, tables and graphical presentations of the available suicide data by age, sex, and race are presented. This compilation of research, clinical, review and demographic materials provides the reader with the most comprehensive and up-to-date reference source on elderly suicide.

To further improve the usefulness of the annotations for empirical works, the table at the end of the introduction lists the sources of data employed in the research investigations as well as the subject populations included. As can be seen, most empirical findings involve the use of official statistics or suicide attempters.

SCOPE OF COVERAGE AND SOURCES

Both the fields of gerontology and suicidology are diverse and include extremely multidisciplinary literatures and professionals. The two fields of study also share greatly expanding research and published works. Professional journals and books in any of the following areas contain written materials on elderly suicide: medicine and health, psychology, sociology, social work, philosophy, psychiatry, anthropology. Gaining accesss to, being aware of, and staying current in the literature from so many disciplines is difficult. The present book includes references from these content areas to provide the reader with the diverse background that encompasses our knowledge and thoughts of elderly suicide.

The only annotated bibliography previously existing on suicide in the elderly was by Marv Miller. He provides, in his book cited above and in the journal Death Education in 1979 (see reference 2-003), brief annotations of 19 empirical articles from 1951 to 1977. The nearly 200 English language empirical and non-empirical works summarized in the present book provide a great expansion of that information. The published works cover the time period from the early 1900s to early 1986, although the majority appeared from around 1970 through the end of 1985. Among the annotated works in Chapters 3 and 4, 82 percent were published since 1970, 62 percent since 1975, 38 percent since 1980, and 9 percent since 1985. The coverage is comprehensive although several sources that only briefly presented a portion of the literature on this topic within coverage of larger concerns (e.g., articles or books on depression in the elderly with a few-paragraph coverage of suicide) have been omitted because they added no information to what was presented here.

The references cited within this book are the result of searches by the two authors of book and journal article reference lists, bibliographies, computer searches and personal searches of indexes, abstract sources, and individual journal issue contents over the period of time the two of us researched and wrote on this topic. Listed below are the index and abstract sources that have been consulted in compiling this book:

Abstracts in Anthropology
Abstracts for Social Workers replaced by: Social Work Research and
    Abstracts
Bulletin of Suicidology
Community Mental Health Review
Current Bibliography of Epidemiology
Current Contents, Social and Behavioral Sciences
Current Literature on Aging
Dissertation Abstracts International
Abstracts on Criminology and Penology replaced by Criminology and
    Penology Abstracts
Excerpta Medica, Section 20: Geriatrics; Section 32: Psychiatry
Gerontological Abstracts
Hospital Literature Index
Index Medicus
International Bibliography of Research in Marriage and the Family
International Bibliography of the Social Sciences--Sociology
International Nursing Index
Marriage and Family Life Review
Nursing and Allied Health Literature Index
Psychological Abstracts

Social Science Citation Index
Social Sciences Index
Sociological Abstracts
Women's Studies Abstracts

    To facilitate the direct and immediate usefulness of this book and
its citations, abbreviations of book and journal titles have been
avoided. For many of the non-English references of Chapter 5 a source
for English abstracts of the citation is included following the
reference itself. The reader wishing to consult a brief summary, for
those that are not annotated here, before securing the original source
itself should find these abstract sources most helpful. The sources of
these abstracts and their abbreviations may be found at the beginning
of Chapter 5 (on page 150). The few abbreviations employed within the
review chapter and the annotations have been defined at the location of
their use.

ACKNOWLEDGMENTS

    This reference book is the result of years of research, reading,
and work into the topic of elderly suicide by both authors. It is our
hope that the materials presented in this work will stimulate interest,
and further research, clinical and preventive efforts on elderly
suicide. Although accuracy in the citations and the information
contained within the annotations have been carefully prepared and
checked, errors may have occurred. We accept full responsibility for
the citations and information appearing here and apologize for any
possible errors and the difficulty they might produce.
    Without a number of individuals this project would not have been
compiled. We wish first to thank our spouses, Raymond Jordan and
Charleen McIntosh, and our children, Cressida Osgood, and Kimberly and
Shawn McIntosh for their patience and indulgence during this endeavor.
Their love and understanding have been extremely important to us.
Dr. John F. Santos of the University of Notre Dame is also acknowledged
for his support and encouragement of the second author. John's
friendship and mentorship both in suicidology and gerontology laid part
of the foundation for this book.
    We wish also to thank a number of people and organizations who
contributed to this volume: our universities and colleagues in the
departments of Psychology at Indiana University at South Bend and
Gerontology at Virginia Commonwealth University/Medical College of
Virginia; the libraries at our universities as well as that of the
University of Notre Dame; the interlibrary loan offices of Indiana
University at South Bend (especially Phyllis Lawrence, Sonja Marshalek,
and Mary Griggs) and Virginia Commonwealth University which processed
the many requests for materials listed here; Rita Handrich, a
Psychology Ph.D. student at Virginia Commonwealth University who wrote
some of the annotations; Susan Griffith, a Virginia Commonwealth
student who helped with some of the library work; our colleagues of
the American Association of Suicidology and the Gerontological Society
of America who have provided feedback on papers presented at their
meetings on the topic of elderly suicide; The Retirement Research
Foundation for the research grants awarded to the second author which

permitted the purchase of a microcomputer used both in research and the generation of this book; and Mary R. Sive of Greenwood Press for her input on the manuscript and its preparation.

The order of authorship was determined by the order in which the two authors entered into the project. Each author contributed equally to the book's contents.

EMPIRICAL INVESTIGATIONS: FROM CHAPTER 4
Data Sources & Subject Populations

COMPLETED SUICIDES		ATTEMPTED SUICIDES
Official Statistics/Records	Interviews with Family	ATTEMPTED SUICIDES
001 003 004 006 009 010 011	007 022 056 065 066	008 012 014 026
016 017 021 025 027 028 029	090	037 038 040 041
030 031 032 033 034 035 039		048 054 073 077
042 045 046 047 057 058 059		078 089 104 113
060 062 063 064 068 069 076		
079 080 082 083 084 085 086		
087 088 091 093 094 095 096		
097 098 099 100 101 102 103		
106 107 113		

COMPLETED SUICIDES		Suicide Notes
Institution/Patient Records	Patient Pop. Follow-up	Suicide Notes
023 026 038 044	018 052 092	016 019 024 043
		049 050

Suicide Ideation Studies	SPC Contacts*	ISDB/ILTB Studies**
002 013 020 053 055 074 075	023 051*** 108	036 067 070 071
081 105		072

Other Studies
005 015 061 109 110 111 112

Note: The numbers listed above refer to the numbering of the references
within Chapter 4. That is, "001" refers to annotation 4-001.

  *: SPC means Suicide Prevention Center.
 **: ISDB means Indirect Self-Destructive Behavior.
     ILTB means Indirect Life-Threatening Behavior.
***: This study investigated those who had completed suicide as well
     as an alive sample of callers to the SPC.

SUICIDE
and the Elderly

1
REVIEW OF THE GERONTOLOGICAL SUICIDE LITERATURE

Suicide represents a major mental health problem in the United States and many other countries. As a cause of death suicide currently (1983 data, National Center for Health Statistics [NCHS], 1985, reference A-007) ranks eighth in the U.S. with nearly 30,000 annual deaths officially classified as suicide. In addition, somewhere between 240,000 and 600,000 Americans attempt suicide annually (Shneidman, 1969; Wolff, 1970b, reference 4-111) and over 5 million living Americans have attempted suicide at some time in their lives (Wekstein, 1979, p. 41). Finally, it is estimated (Shneidman, 1969) that each suicide death intimately affects at least 6 family members or friends ("survivors victims" or "survivors of suicide"). There are undoubtedly millions of survivors currently in the U.S. (Andress & Corey, 1978) and their rolls increase by at least 180,000 annually. These estimates and figures clearly demonstrate the importance of suicidal behavior and the need for both attention and preventive efforts.

DEMOGRAPHIC FACTORS AND SUICIDE AMONG THE ELDERLY

Two dramatic changes have taken place in U.S. (and many other countries') suicide rates by age. First, there has been a large increase in suicide among young people (especially those aged 15–24) in recent years which has received tremendous attention among professionals and the public. The second change has been at least equally as dramatic but has largely been ignored or overlooked although it has occurred among an even higher risk group. Over a longer period of time than that in which youth suicide increases have taken place, suicide rates for the aged have declined markedly (see the tables and figures in Chapter 6 for official U.S. suicide data by age over time and for various demographic factors; A graph of similar declines in England and Wales may be found in Morgan, 1979, p. 16).

An important point to note is that, despite sizeable increases in suicide rates for the young and declines for the old, the elderly remain clearly at higher risk for suicide. For example, in 1983, U.S. suicide rates were 12.1 for the nation, 11.9 for 15–24–year–olds, and 19.2 for those over 65 (based on data in NCHS, 1985, reference A-007). Thus, the highest rates of suicide by age are found not among the young but among the elderly. This observation has been true as long as official suicide data have been kept by the U.S. government (see the tables in Chapter 6) and is accurate for most other countries as well (Shulman, 1978, reference 3-055).

This chapter will focus predominantly on explanations and preventive measures with respect to the high suicide rates of the old. Before doing so, however, explanations for the declines that have occurred as well as the high risk subgroups within the elderly population will be considered. White males are at highest risk for suicide as are the very old (over 75 years of age; McIntosh, 1984, reference 4-059; see also Kastenbaum, 1985). Male rates of suicide increase and peak in old age while female rates increase until middle age (mid-40s to mid-50s) and decline thereafter. Female suicide rates are generally lower than those for males at all ages, and particularly so in old age (see McIntosh & Jewell, 1986). Suicide rates for whites in the U.S. increase with age and peak in old age while those for nonwhites peak in young adulthood (generally in the 20s or early 30s) and decline thereafter (there are, however, specific racial/ethnic group differences, see McIntosh, 1985, and McIntosh & Santos, 1981, reference 4-062). As will be detailed later in this chapter, in addition to whites and males, other high risk geriatric groups include the widowed, those who have experienced recent losses, those with physical illnesses and intractable pain, and those who have undergone various status changes.

Reasons for the decline in elderly suicide are not apparent and there is inadequate information to explain these changes (McIntosh, 1983), since few writers or investigators have focused on this issue. It is unlikely that suicide prevention center efforts have contributed greatly to the changes because the old rarely utilize these facilities (see e.g., Atkinson, 1971, reference 4-005). The old typically represent only 1%-2% of the caseloads of suicide prevention centers (see e.g., McIntosh, Hubbard, & Santos, 1981, reference 3-070). Busse (1974, p. 221) suggested that antidepressants and increases in economic security and health care are possible factors in the decline.

Research has provided at least partial answers to some of the possible contributing factors. Although the rise in the elderly population as a whole does not appear to be closely associated with their decreased suicide rates (Holinger & Offer, 1982, reference 4-033), the increasing number of women compared to men in older age categories has been significantly related to the decline (McIntosh, Hubbard, & Santos, 1980). As will be seen below, women are a low risk group for suicide at all ages (and especially in old age) while men are generally a high risk group both overall and particularly in old age. As the total aged population has come to include larger proportions of women, the effect has been to contribute to the decrease in elderly suicide rates. In addition, most of the declines in elderly suicide have been among males and this has also accelerated the decline over the influence that might be attributable to increasing numbers of females alone.

Another factor that has influenced the decreasing suicide rates in old age is economic in nature. Marshall (1978, reference 4-058) found a significant correlation between decreased suicide rates for white males 65-74 years of age and improved economic status among the group. The impact on the most important elderly group with respect to suicide rates (i.e., old white males, McIntosh, 1984, reference 4-059) has had a major influence on the decline among the elderly as a whole.

From a demographic standpoint, the declines in suicide rates have been noted for both males and females but clearly much more for males. The declines for the aged as a whole, therefore, have been produced primarily by those decreases among elderly men. The small declines among aged women have not greatly affected the overall aged rates. Likewise, the elderly declines have been almost exclusively among whites. Nonwhite elderly suicide rates are extremely low and have changed little over time. With respect to the various age groups which comprise the old population, declines have occurred for all aged groups but have been slightly larger among the young-old (65-74 or 55-74) than among the old-old (75+). Within the old-old population, greater declines in rates have been observed for the 75-84 population than for those 85 and above.   Once again, the declines for both the young-old and old-old have been predominantly a white male phenomenon (McIntosh, 1984, reference 4-059).   Whatever the ultimate explanation for the decline, successive cohorts of elderly have become increasingly lower risks for suicide than were their predecessors. As will be seen in the discussion of cohort analyses, however, such a trend may not continue as the currently younger cohorts, who seem to be at higher risks than their predecessors at all ages, reach older ages. Although the old are lower risks today than in the past, however, it should be kept in mind that they remain the highest risk age group for suicide.

From the previous discussion it is clear that, compared to other age groups, the old are most "at risk" for committing suicide, and certain categories of older individuals are more vulnerable than others.   Compared to younger individuals, older adults openly communicate their suicidal intent less frequently (Jarvis & Boldt, 1980, reference 4-034; Kopell, 1977, reference 3-020) use more violent and lethal methods (McIntosh & Santos, 1985-86, reference 4-063), and less often attempt suicide as a means of gaining attention or to cry for help (Pasquali & Bucher, 1981, reference 5-063; Summa, 1977, reference 5-082; Sendbuehler, 1977, reference 3-051).   All of these factors increase the risk of death for the old. In spite of the fact that older adults´are particularly at risk with respect to suicide, in this society we have paid much more attention to other age groups, especially teenagers and young adults (see for example, the bibliographies on youth suicide, McIntosh, 1981a, 1984a, 107 and 35 pages, respectively, compared to those for the elderly, McIntosh, 1981b, 1984b, references 2-001, 37 pages, and 2-002, 10 pages, respectively). We have tended to place a fairly low priority on saving the lives of our old.

In this part of the chapter we will examine some major factors in elderly suicide, as well as various explanations--drawn from sociology, psychology and other disciplines--which have been offered to explain the high rate of suicide among the old and why certain groups of elderly are more vulnerable. We will also discuss recognition and assessment of suicidal risk and prevention and intervention. Finally we will discuss the ethical issues surrounding elderly suicide and offer suggestions for future areas of research and study.

FACTORS AND EXPLANATIONS

The Cultural Context

Cowgill and Holmes (1972) developed a cross-societal theory of aging demonstrating a strong relationship between level of modernization in society (based on level of technology, degree of urbanization, rate of social change, and degree of Westernization) and status of the aged. They concluded that in Western technologically advanced societies the aged are devalued and hold less power, status, and economic control than in less advanced societies. Their theory gained further support from Palmore and Manton's (1974) cross-cultural study in 31 countries, which demonstrated that the status of the aged is lower in more modernized cultures. Suicide rates of the aged are highest in urban, industrialized countries, such as the United States (Quinney, 1965)

Rosow (1967) argues that the relative position of the aged in any society is governed by six institutional factors: (1) their ownership of property and control over the opportunities of the young, (2) their command of strategic knowledge and skills, (3) strong religiosity and sacred traditions, (4) strong kinship and extended family bonds in a communal or Gemeinschaft-type of social organization, (5) a low productivity economy, and (6) high mutual dependence and reciprocal aid among members (p. 9). In American society, according to Rosow, the aged suffer a loss of status position on all these institutional dimensions.

American society highly values youth and beauty, productivity, progress, speed, and independence. In his classic study of American society, Robin Williams (1970) concluded that occupational success is not just one life goal among others in American society, but is the outstanding trait of American culture. Mizruchi's (1964) work further confirms the emphasis on work and success in our society. Retired from participation in the occupational role, the elderly may suffer a severe loss of status, role, and power in our society, as well as a loss of income.

Societies that place a high value on age have low suicide rates in their older populations (Quinney, 1965) When societies modernize and industrialize, the rates of elderly self-destruction increase (e.g., Hong Kong, Yap, 1963, reference 4-113; Stack, 1982a, reference 4-097, studied 45 cultures; Mizruchi, 1982) Seiden (1983, reference 3-050) recently noted that "As cultures become less traditional, when age is no longer seen as a pathway to wisdom, when extended families fly to the wind, when people are considered interchangeable parts, when progress is highly valued, the suicide rates of the elderly will rise" (p. 5). Mizruchi (1982) suggests that a numerical surplus population segment can become superfluous and therefore structurally disadvantaged if opportunities to participate in society are absent and people are held in terminal rather than transitional positions. This situation is more likely to occur in more modernized societies. Support for this notion comes from Atchley's (1980, reference 4-004) study of suicide in various societies. Atchley found that societies that have high chronic disease rates also have high suicide rates, especially among those 65 and over.

The elderly in this society are often viewed as useless, dependent, nonproductive, and a burden to be borne by younger members of the society. They are "over the hill, down the drain, out to pasture, fading fast" (Butler, 1975, p. 2). They are often the victims of ageism or negative stereotyping. Images of aging found in books, cartoons, well-known jokes and sayings, and the media present a picture of the elderly as sexless and senile, grumpy and cranky, rigid and conservative in their values and thinking, wrinkled and toothless (Butler, 1975; Troll, Israel, & Israel, 1977). As Lillian Troll suggests, the stereotype of the elderly woman in this country portrays her as "poor," "dumb," and "ugly" (e.g., Troll et al., 1977). The elderly in this country are advised to buy cream to cover up "those ugly age spots and wrinkles," to join health and figure spas, and to try all sorts of diets to "keep that youthful figure." Hair dyes to "get rid of that ugly gray," dentures and tooth polish to "recapture that youthful smile," and tonics and pills to "feel young and look young again" are also available.

In our youth-oriented, production-minded society the aged are devalued. Their skills become obsolete in the face of technological change. Their wisdom and experience, gained from years of living, are not valued by many in the next generations who confront a different world from the one in which their parents and grandparents lived.

Another subtle indication of the devaluation of the old can be seen in a recent statistic that has been included in governmental publications on suicide. The Centers for Disease Control (1985, p. 356) stated that in 1980 "suicide accounted for a loss of some 619,533 years of potential life lost for individuals between the ages of 1 and 65 years" (emphasis added). This statistic was "calculated by multiplying the number of suicides in each 5-year age category by the difference between age 65 and the midpoint for the 1-14 year age category." The implication seems to be that those over age 65 either had no or little potential life to lose by committing suicide. In a society that values youth and productivity, it is a small move from "potential life lost" to "potential productive life lost." Since the old are most often not contributing directly through active work roles, their older years are frequently seen as unproductive for society. The message that may be given by such a statistic and the way it is derived is that young suicide is more tragic than an old person's suicide. Indeed, a study by Cameron (1972, reference 4-015) found that all age groups were less opposed to suicide when it was committed by an old person.

How do the elderly view themselves in such a culture? Presumably, when all of the diets and pills and creams and cosmetics fail, the elderly are forced to see themselves as old. Indeed, many accept the negative cultural images, and consequently their self-esteem and self-concept suffer (Birren & Sloane, 1980; Lehr, 1981). These individuals may feel that they are useless, unwanted, unneeded, and unloved in such a culture. Ageism and negative cultural images have been noted as a source of stress in late life (Lehr, 1979; Loether, 1975; Payne, 1975, reference 3-039).

The Sociological Perspective

Although earlier writers had reported a relationship between suicide rates and various variables, the first well-known sociological study of suicide was conducted in 1897 by Emile Durkheim. Durkheim's (1897/1951, reference 3-014) Suicide has exerted a major influence on sociology as a discipline and served as a blueprint for later sociological studies of suicide in particular (for contemporary research based on Durkheim's theoretical notions, see McIntosh, 1985, reference 2-007, pp. 44-45). Durkheim sought explanations for variations in the suicide rate in terms of the degree to which people are integrated in the society and the extent to which their conduct is regulated (Giddens, 1971). He derived two major propositions: (1) that the suicide rate varies inversely with the degree of integration of the group, and (2) that the suicide rate varies inversely with the degree of normative regulation.

Regarding the former, suicide varies with the strength of bonds between the person and the groups with which the person is affiliated. Thus, not only are persons more vulnerable to suicide if they are too weakly integrated into groups, which provide meaning and control over their lives, but excessive integration also increases their proclivity to suicide. What Durkheim called integration has something to do with a person's social ties to the larger group, with a person's level of meaningful interaction with other members of the larger social group, and with that person's degree of social "belongingness."

In his famous typology of suicide, Durkheim describes two types resulting from man's level of integration into society. He postulated that persons who are deeply and intimately involved with others in various social groups should be low suicide risks. He consequently found the unmarried to have the highest rate of suicide. He identified the type of suicide that results from lack of integration as "egoistic." According to Durkheim, the stronger the forces throwing one onto one's own resources, the greater the likelihood of egoistic suicide. Durkheim classified suicide among the aged as "egoistic." He proposed that suicide increased with age because society as a moral force begins to recede from the person, in terms of both goals and commitments, as the person ages and withdraws from various roles and positions. The older individual is less integrated into and less dependent upon society.

Building on the early work of Durkheim, Rosow (1967) suggested that the elderly tend to be less integrated into society due to (1) their removal and withdrawal from certain organizational contexts and associated roles, thereby weakening their ties to mediating structures, such as work, voluntary associations, and like organizations, and (2) the contraction of their intimate social world, which results from relocation, incapacitation, and death of friends and peers.

Not only are the elderly more likely to commit "egoistic suicide" because of their lack of integration into formal and informal social groups, they are also more likely to commit "anomic suicide." As Rosow (1967) and Neugarten (1968a) point out, our culture does not provide older members with definitions and meaningful norms, so older persons are left to structure the "aged role" for themselves, with no clear prescriptions as to the appropriate behavior. Durkheim refers to this condition as "anomie."

Old age, unlike other stages in the life cycle, is also the first stage of life with systematic status loss, as Rosow (1967) aptly points out. All other statuses, from childhood through adolescence and full maturity, are normally marked by steady social acquisitions of power, prestige, and rewards. When people enter the later stages of life and assume the aged role, however, for the first time loss of status is experienced. They now realize that the life goals they set for themselves may never be attained, as the resources for achieving them dwindle before their eyes. They also realize that the time they have left may not allow for the realization of goals or the life changes that might be necessary to attain such goals (e.g., Neugarten, 1968b). Such a realization may lead to feelings of despair by the elderly rather than feeling that one's life has been meaningful and contributed to society (Erikson, 1963).

Another factor producing a greater probability of suicide in the elderly results from the changes in expectations associated with stages in the life cycle. Norms of achievement, which operated throughout the earlier stages, now give way to relatively amorphous norms of ascription as the bases of judging the behavior of the elderly. Persons pass into a stage in which they become socially defined as old, in which the basis for judgement shifts from criteria of performance to those of age, regardless of accomplishment (Rosow, 1973).

In sum, older age status appears to be accompanied by decreasing opportunity to function as an effective member of society and by an increasing inability to achieve life goals. This pattern may be expected to result in despair, demoralization, and uneasiness.

Some older individuals are less integrated and less constrained by society than are others. We would expect that such individuals will be the most prone to commit suicide in later life. Differences in suicide rates by gender, race, and marital status can be explained using such a perspective.

In his book, Durkheim reported that suicide varied by age and gender. Most notable was the markedly high ratio, 3:1, for suicides of men compared to those of women. Durkheim recognized that participation in the family represented one of the most important ties among society's members. He suggested that the state of marriage and membership in a family integrate societal members by exerting a regulative force on them and by acting as a stimulant to intensive interpersonal relations that draw the members into firm and meaningful union, thus providing some degree of immunity, the "coefficient of preservation" against suicide. Durkheim explained higher rates of suicide among widows and widowers as due to "domestic anomie," that is, a deregulation of behavior resulting from the spouse's death. He also viewed the loss of the spouse as weakening the familial integration of the individual. Thus, the suicide of widows and widowers may be referred to as both "anomic" and "egoistic." Berardo (1968, 1970) similarly describes the situation of the widowed as vague and unstructured, lacking clear guidelines for behavior, and lacking supportive interaction with friends, kin, and coworkers. Two other followers of Durkheim, Henry and Short (1954), have explained suicide in terms of the weakening of the relational system constituted by marriage, and Bock (1972, reference 4-009) points out that "marriage not only integrates the individual into a close and meaningful association but also regulates him by requiring him to take the other person into account in activities and decisions" (p. 72). The loss of a spouse represents the loss of a major social role in the institution of the family, as well as the loss of a sexual partner, confidant, companion and friend. Such an important social and emotional loss often leaves the individual sad and lonely, feeling life is meaningless and empty. Research has consistently revealed higher suicide rates for widowed individuals, especially in the first two years following the death of a spouse (Gardner, Bahn, & Mack, 1964, reference 4-026; Gubrium, 1974; Kopell, 1977, reference 3-020; MacMahon & Pugh, 1965, reference 4-056; Maris, 1969; Payne, 1975, reference 3-039; Resnik & Cantor, 1970, reference 3-045; Wenz, 1976, reference 4-102).

Durkheim's classic explanation for the greater proportion of suicides among widowers, as compared to widows, was that men derive more from marriage than women (Durkheim, 1897/1951, reference 3-014). The elderly widower is likely to be the most vulnerable to suicide (Berardo, 1967, 1968, 1970; Bock, 1972, reference 4-009; Gubrium, 1974). Several explanations have been offered for the increased vulnerability of elderly male widowers. After some pioneering studies, Berardo suggested more than ten years ago that the elderly widower suffers doubly because he loses not only his role in the family system but his role in the occupational sphere as well. He also pointed out that in our society the woman has assumed the responsibility for integrating the kinship group and maintaining contacts with friends and relatives over the years. As a result, she has the support of the kinship group when her husband dies, but the elderly widower is left totally alone. The elderly male widower is among the most socially isolated individuals in our society. He has fewer relatives and kin living nearby, participates less with family and friends, and is less involved in formal organizations and the community than his female widowed counterpart.

Elderly males in our society often suffer another major loss in late life, loss of their work role. Powell (1970) notes that the male is primarily integrated into American society through the occupational role. If one accepts Powell's assumption that occupation constitutes a basis of status integration for members of American society,

particularly for men, then one   must conclude that the absence or
deprivation of occupation results in loss of status integration or loss
of status.   Accordingly, many retired men may be viewed as living in a
condition of anomie.   Many researchers have noted the   increased
vulnerability to suicide of the retired male (Breed & Huffine, 1979,
reference 3-007; Farberow & Moriwaki, 1975, reference 4-023; Kopell,
1977, reference 3-020;   Miller, 1979, reference 3-027;   Peretti &
Wilson, 1978-79, reference 4-075; Sainsbury, 1968, reference 4-086;
Strahan, 1980, reference 3-058).

Blau (1956) has offered an explanation for the dramatically higher
rates of suicide among elderly males, reflecting the sociological
perspective known as the role theory perspective. In her work, Blau
noted the negative effect of cumulative role loss: the more social
roles lost, the greater the negative impact. Elderly males lose their
roles in two major social institutions in society: work and the
family. The male may have relied strongly on "his occupation and
co-workers earlier in life for social and personal identity, and
retirement may have forced him to depend more heavily on his spouse for
personal social significance. Under these conditions, her death would
have meant even greater isolation from kin and community groups" (Blau,
1956, p. 62).   Townsend (1968) has referred to this   change   or
discontinuity in social engagements, experienced most acutely by male
widowers who have lost roles in the work and family world, as
"desolation."

Compared to black males and white females, aged white males in
American society suffer the most severe loss of social status and
position, power, and money. This status loss represents one possible
explanation for their dramatically higher rates of suicide. Breed
(1963), Maris (1969), McIntosh and Santos (1981, reference 4-062), and
Powell (1970) have all related the high suicide rates of elderly white
males to the severe loss of status, power, money, and role
relationships formerly provided by participation in work.   By
comparison, women generally and minority males, two groups that
traditionally have held lower status positions in our society, have
less to lose upon retirement than white males and thus tend to display
lower rates of suicide than white males. Maris (1969), McIntosh and
Santos (1981, reference 4-062), and Seiden (1981, reference 3-049) all
attribute the lower rate of suicide among older blacks, as compared to
older whites, to the greater degree of external constraint imposed upon
blacks and to their more intense involvement in family, church, and
other social relational systems.   Seiden (1981, reference 3-049) argues
that elderly blacks are wanted and needed in the family system,
sometimes due to economic necessity, but also because old age is
respected by blacks, and they therefore feel they belong and are useful
and productive.   According to Seiden, the intense support networks and
strong human relationships that characterize the black community
protect elderly blacks against suicide.

The Psychological Perspective

Negative cultural stereotypes of the old, coupled with their loss
of important social roles in the world of family, work, and community,

with the concomitant weakening of social integration and regulation, are major sources of stress in late life. In addition to social losses, the elderly suffer many other losses including: loss of health, impaired vision and/or hearing, loss of mobility, financial loss, loss of home and possessions, loss of independence, and cognitive loss and mental impairment. These losses result in stress at a time in life when the individual is least able to resist and cope with stress. These losses, and the stress suffered from them, often result in feelings of depression and despair (Miller, 1979, reference 3-027; Osgood, 1985b, reference 3-034; Stenback, 1980, reference 3-056).

Depression is the most common functional psychiatric disorder of late life (Blazer, 1982; Pfeiffer, 1977; Salzman & Shader, 1979). Depression, the major factor in late life suicide, underlies two-thirds of the suicides in the elderly (Gurland & Cross, 1983). Batchelor (1957, reference 3-003) noted that at least 80% of all suicidal old people were depressed. In another statement Batchelor went so far as to suggest that "all suicidal old people . . . are depressed" (p. 291). Depression in late life has been related to other factors besides loss and stress. Senescent changes in the organism, particularly evolutional changes in the brain and nervous and endocrine systems and accelerated cerebral tissue loss, are factors in the development of depression in late life (Meier-Ruge, 1975; Gaitz & Varner, 1980; Birren & Sloane, 1980). Depression may also result from some viral infections and from Parkinson's disease (Birren & Sloane, 1980; Gerner, 1979; Robins, 1976; Wilson, 1976). Organic brain syndromes have been noted in association with nonfatal suicide attempts in old age by some researchers (e.g., Kiroboe, 1951, reference 4-038; Sendbuehler & Goldstein, 1977, reference 4-089).

Three major factors have been recognized as contributing to depression and suicide among the aged (and those of other ages): haplessness, helplessness, and hopelessness. Lowered self-concept and self-esteem contribute to the haplessness and self-hatred of the aged (Pavkov, 1982, reference 3-038). Seligman (1975, 1976) defines helplessness as a state in which individuals experience an inability to control significant life events and suggests that it is the core of all depression. The aged are then most susceptible to helplessness, according to Seligman, because they have experienced the greatest loss of control. Schulz (1976) similarly argues that loss of job, income, physical health, work, and childbearing roles results in increased helplessness and depression in the aged.

Helplessness and hopelessness often go hand in hand and can result in suicidal behavior in the aged. Karl Menninger (1938), who has exerted a major influence on the study of depression and suicide in the aged, postulated that suicide results from three wishes: the wish to kill, the wish to be killed, and the wish to die. He characterized suicides of the elderly as a result of the wish to die (studies of suicide notes among various age groups support this contention, see e.g., Farberow & Shneidman, 1957/1970, reference 4-024). In emphasizing the wish to die as a major motive in elderly suicide, Menninger identified hopelessness as a major contributing factor. Farber (1968) similarly conceived of suicide among the aged as a desperate response to hopeless and intolerable life situations, when he wrote "Suicide occurs when there appears to be no available path that will lead to a tolerable existence. . . . It is when the life interest is one of despairing hopelessness that suicide occurs" (p. 17). Farber defines hope as the relationship between a sense of personal competence and life-threatening events. Those who have analyzed suicide notes of individuals of various ages have found that the elderly express a sense of hopelessness and "psychological exhaustion" in their notes (Cath, 1965; Darbonne, 1969, reference 4-019; Farberow & Shneidman, 1957/1970, reference 4-024). They are tired of life and tired of living. They have just given up. The sense of rage and anger which is often expressed by younger people in their notes is absent from the notes of older individuals.

Other factors that increase vulnerability to suicide—many of them secondary to depression—include bereavement, diagnosis of cancer or other terminal illness, a major life move, or a serious argument or flare-up with a family member or close friend.

ASSESSMENT AND PREVENTION

The Role of Physicians

Physicians are most often the ones to whom the desperate elderly turn. Over 75% of the elderly who commit suicide see a physician shortly before the act (Foster & Burke, 1985, reference 3-015; Litman, Curphey, Shneidman, Farberow, & Tabachnick, 1963; Miller, 1977, 1979, references 3-026 & 3-027, respectively). Sainsbury (1963, 1968, references 4-085 & 4-086, respectively) found in his study of geriatric suicides in London that 70% of them had seen a doctor within a month before taking their own lives. Marv Miller (1976) similarly found that 76% of the elderly male suicides he studied had seen a physician within the month prior to their death. The important role of the physician in preventing elderly suicide thus cannot be overemphasized. In order to accurately assess suicidal intentions in their older patients, physicians should be aware of the demographic and personal background factors and life style characteristics that predispose one to commit suicide.

The physician must also become "depression conscious," to use the term employed by Bennett (1967, reference 3-004). Many writers in the area have noted the importance of accurate diagnosis and treatment of depression in preventing suicide in the older individual (Chaisson, 1981; Foster & Burke, 1985, reference 3-015; Friedel, 1982; Kopell, 1977, reference 3-020; Melville & Blazer, 1985; Payne, 1975, reference 3-039; Patterson, Abrahams, & Baker, 1974, reference 3-037; Pfeiffer & Busse, 1973, reference 3-041).

Accurate diagnosis of depression depends on good listening skills and taking the time to notice the signs of depression, as well as various laboratory tests which can be performed. By taking a little time to listen to the elderly patient, paying particular attention to the tone of the voice, handshake, facial expression, dress and personal grooming, and mood state, the physician might be alerted that something is seriously wrong, and that something is not just a medical problem. Various standardized instruments to assess depression have been developed and can be administered to older individuals to aid the physician in making a diagnosis (Beck, 1967; Hamilton, 1960; Zung, 1965).

Two psychoendocrinologic tests of research interest are now being used clinically to diagnose depression. The TRH stimulation test involves testing the level of thyrotropin (TSH) secreted by the body in response to infusion of thyrotropin-releasing hormone (TRH). This response has been found to be blunted in 25 to 56% of patients with major depression and, in addition, is abnormal in some alcoholics, manics, and patients with anorexia nervosa (Loosen & Prange, 1982). Dexamethasone Suppression Test (DST) involves testing the body's response to a synthetic steroid that, when taken by mouth, usually supresses secretion of cortisol for up to 24 hours (Carroll et al., 1981). After baseline studies, the drug is given orally at 11 P.M. The next day, two or three serial determinations are made of serum cortisol. Many studies have confirmed that up to 50% of seriously depressed patients will have test values elevated above the normal of 5 mcgms/ml. Moreover, successful somatic therapy of these same patients will usually result in a return of the test response to normal. Thus, both recovery and relapse can be monitored by following the DST. The DST has been recommended by Melville and Blazer (1985) and Friedel (1982).

Another important new diagnostic study emerging from the research sector into clinical practice is the sleep electroencephalogram (EEG). Disruptions of the sleep-wake cycle, including sleep continuity, rapid eye movement (REM) activity, density and latency, are characteristic of several states, including normal old age, depression, and dementia. REM sleep is one of the elements of normal sleep, occurring several times during the night and is characterized by a specific pattern on the sleep EEG. The period of REM latency is the amount of time that passes from the onset of sleep until the first REM period begins. In normal adults, REM latency is 60 minutes or more, however, it may be reduced to 30-50 minutes or less in persons suffering from major depressive illness (Coble, Kupfer, & Shaw, 1981). In addition to increased REM activity and density, depressed subjects often have numerous waking periods. Recent studies have indicated that depressives show more disturbances on sleep EEG recordings than normals and that the severities of the disturbances and depression are positively correlated (Spiker, Coble, Cofsky, Foster, & Kupfer, 1980).

Treatment of depression in the elderly is a major factor in suicide prevention. Pharmacological intervention using tricyclic antidepressants or monoamine oxidase inhibitors has been very effective (Borson & Veith, 1985; Chaisson, 1981; Cassano, Maggini, & Akiskai, 1983; Friedel, 1982) as has electroconvulsive therapy (Borson & Veith, 1985; Bidder, 1981; Chaisson, 1981; Kendell, 1981; Malloy, Small, Miller, Milstein, & Stout, 1982).

Various other treatment modalities such as psychotherapy or other "talk therapies," and involvement in various supportive therapies, which will be discussed in more detail later in this section, have also proven effective in combatting depression in late life. Physicians and other practitioners working with the elderly should become familiar with these treatment modalities. Physicians should also be aware of psychiatric and other community services available to deal with the depressed elderly and make referrals, when appropriate (Bennett, 1967, reference 3-004; Berdes, 1978, reference 3-006; Payne, 1975, reference 3-039).

Reading Suicidal Clues and Assessing Lethality Potential

Many suicidal elderly individuals give clues before they commit suicide. In his in-depth investigation of 301 completed suicides, Miller (1978b, reference 4-066) discovered that 60% of them gave verbal or behavioral clues to their self-inflicted deaths. Robins, West, and Murphy (1977, reference 4-081) similarly found in their study that two-thirds of those who eventually killed themselves had previously communicated their intent to commit suicide. When clues to suicide are encountered in the old, it is particularly important to respond because they may give fewer clues than other groups and they seem more intent to die (see e.g., Farberow & Shneidman, 1957/1970, reference 4-024). In addition, we may have to combat a belief "that there can be [no] such a thing as premature death in old age." People may feel that "it is all right for the aged to die. It is their task, their responsibility" (Kastenbaum, 1972, p. 123). Ignoring clues by the old may simply reinforce their feelings of worthlessness and "duty" to die (Lesnoff-Caravaglia, 1983, reference 3-021).

Shneidman (1965, reference 3-053) has classified clues as verbal, behavioral, situational, and syndromatic. Pavkov (1982, reference 3-038), Osgood (1985b, reference 3-034), Foster and Burke (1985, reference 3-015) and others have all provided checklists of the types of clues to look for in suicidal elderly individuals. Many of the signs of depression in the elderly are also clues to impending suicidal behavior.

The following examples of clues are provided by Osgood (1985b, reference 3-034).

Verbal Clues
- I am going to kill myself.
- I'm going to commit suicide.
- I'm going to end it all.
- I want to end it all.
- I just want out.
- You would be better off without me.

Behavioral Clues
- donating body to a medical school
- purchasing a gun
- stockpiling pills
- putting personal and business affairs in order
- making or changing a will
- taking out insurance or changing beneficiaries

- making funeral plans
- giving away money and/or possessions
- changes in behavior, especially episodes of screaming or hitting, throwing things or failure to get along with family, friends, or peers
- suspicious behavior, for example, going out at odd times of the day or night, waving or kissing goodbye (if not characteristic)
- sudden interest or disinterest in church and religion
- scheduling of appointment with doctor for no apparent physical cause or very shortly after the last visit to the doctor
- loss of physical skills, general confusion, or loss of understanding, judgment, or memory

The most important steps in evaluation of lethality potential are ascertaining first the existence of a suicide plan and then determining the lethality, availability, and accessibility of the method of self-destruction specified in the plan. The suicide plan can be defined as "those suicidal ideations or conceptualizations of suicide and the ways and means of suicide that can lead to the final act of taking his/her life" (Hatton, Valente, & Rink, 1977, p. 52). There are four criteria to assess in order to determine the seriousness of a suicidal plan: (1) method (has the individual decided on pills, hanging, or some other method?), (2) availability (is the method available? easily accessible? possible to gain access to?), (3) specificity (is the method concrete and definite? is the plan all worked out regarding time, place, and other specific details?), and (4) lethality (is shooting, the most lethal method, the one chosen?).

To determine the extent and lethality potential of the suicide plan, the practitioner must ask a series of direct, straightforward questions. Many physicians and other caregivers still believe that asking directly about suicidal thoughts, feelings, or intentions will encourage the individual to commit suicide. In reality, the opposite is true. Not asking encourages suicide. When asked, most individuals readily discuss their suicidal feelings and intentions and are glad to be able to share their thoughts with someone who cares enough to ask. They can achieve great relief by bringing their suicidal intentions out into the open and sharing their tortured "secret" (Hatton et al., 1977; Pavkov, 1982, reference 3-038; Shneidman, 1965, reference 3-053).

The questions asked may be general ones, such as "How is your life going?" If the answers to such questions suggest possible suicidal thoughts or intentions, more specific questions should then be asked. For example:
- Are you thinking of suicide?
- Have you worried about suicide?
- Do you wish you could end it all?
- Do you feel you would be better off dead?

A friendly, matter-of-fact tone of voice should be used. Questions that are "minimizing" or "negatively prompting" should be avoided (Oliven, 1951). Such inappropriate questions include:

        - Just a routine question, but are you thinking of suicide?
        - You aren't thinking of anything like that, but just let me
          ask you . . . ?

A qualified denial of suicidal intent usually indicates a low lethality
potential. A hedging reply ("Who knows?"), a flood of self-accusations
("I'm not fit to live."), or an admission of intent signals high
lethality potential. If such answers are given, direct questions
regarding the suicide plan are essential.

    To ascertain the details of the suicide plan, the practitioner
must ask what particular method, if any, has been chosen. If the
method is shooting, the practitioner should ask directly if the elderly
individual has a gun or can easily get one. Shooting, hanging, jumping
from high places, and cutting are among the most lethal methods.
Taking poison or analgesic or soporific substances is a less lethal
method. If the individual has a definite plan and has chosen a lethal
and available method, steps should be taken immediately to protect him
or her. Finding someone to stay with the person, prescribing
antidepressants, or even hospitalization may be necessary.

Education

    According to Osgood (1985b, reference 3-034), education is a major
key to suicide prevention in late life. Such education, focused on the
symptoms of depression and the warning signs of suicide, should involve
not only the elderly themselves but also the personnel who serve the
elderly, and should be included in public education about the elderly
and aging.

    In addition to general education concerned with the aging process
and how to cope with growing older, the elderly need to be educated
about depression and suicide. The symptoms of depression and the
warning signals of suicide should be recognized by the elderly
individual who is properly informed. The elderly should be aware not
only of the symptoms of depression and of ways to recognize suicidal
thoughts and impulses in themselves, they should also be taught that
depression is treatable and that suicide can be prevented. The
vulnerable elderly in particular should be educated regarding the kind
and variety of help available to them in their community--the
psychological and mental health services, the support groups, and other
church, community, and social services that can provide aid and
guidance. The media, churches, doctors, nurses, social workers,
pharmacists, workers in adult day care centers, and other caregivers
who come in contact with the aged can all play roles in such education.

    Miller (1979, reference 3-027) has identified "retirement shock"
as a major precipitating factor in suicide of elderly males. Education
and preparation for retirement can clearly play important roles in
easing the transition from worker to retiree. Indeed, research has
documented the positive effects of preretirement training on adjustment
to retirement (Atchley, 1976; Glamser & DeJong, 1975; Palmore, 1982).
The elderly also need general leisure education in order to develop
what Tedrick (1982) has referred to as "leisure competency." Many

older individuals have large blocks of time on their hands and no knowledge of how to meaningfully fill the hours. In a recent large-scale survey of older adults conducted by the American Association of Retired Persons (AARP, 1980), older people identified the problem of how to use the increased amount of leisure time as their third most significant problem, following health and finances. Older persons who are educated on the value, meaning, and proper use of leisure time are more likely to acquire leisure competency. Older people who have acquired leisure competency have clarified their values on the use of discretionary time, have a knowledge of available leisure resources and services, and have developed skills and appreciations that lead to enjoyment of participation in selected areas (Tedrick, 1982).

Major emphasis should be placed on educating physicians and other personnel in health and mental health fields and those in occupations that serve the elderly, concerning the processes of aging, thereby making them better prepared to meet the needs of the elderly. Medical, nursing, and other professional schools should include courses about aging (and suicide) in their curricula. Inservice and on-the-job training programs should be offered for practitioners already working in the field. These programs should be focused on dispelling existing myths about suicide, aging and the old.

Physicians, clergy, law enforcement personnel, social workers, and other geriatricians also need to be educated regarding the symptoms of depression in late life and the clues and warning signs of suicide in the elderly. Graduate and professional schools can play a major role in providing such education. The media can help by providing adequate information to service providers working with elderly clients.

Like the service providers and the elderly, the public needs to be educated particularly about the symptoms of depression and the warning signals of suicide in the aged as well as community services that deal with the suicidal and elderly. When properly informed, family members, friends, and neighbors are in an ideal position to save the life of a potentially suicidal elderly individual.

Accurate Case Finding and Active Outreach

It is a well-established fact that suicide prevention centers are not utilized by the elderly (Farberow & Moriwaki, 1975, reference 4-023; McIntosh et al., 1981, reference 3-070; Tuckman, 1970). The vulnerable elderly are also not likely to call social service agencies. More aggressive means of case finding and a more active outreach are needed to reach the lonely, isolated, depressed, or suicide-prone elderly. Such persons must be actively sought, using tips from doctors, pharmacists, staff people at adult day care centers, the clergy, the police, and others who come in contact with them. Health departments, welfare offices, social security offices, and geriatric screening programs can also provide relevant leads and information. McIntosh et al. (1981, reference 3-070) suggest establishing separate hot lines for the elderly, setting up special centers to reach the troubled elderly, using other seniors in a sort of "buddy system" to reach those who are vulnerable, and establishing community-based outreach programs to find the suicide-prone elderly. In all these efforts, early case finding is a key to suicide prevention.

Services and Therapies

The prevention of suicide among the elderly may ultimately depend on societal changes--for example, the satisfaction of basic economic needs and the reduction of poverty among the elderly, improved nutrition and health care delivery, improved transportation, more and better psychological and mental health services, more flexible retirement policies, allowances for elderly individuals to continue working, at least part-time, better preparation for retirement, provision of more and safer housing, increased opportunities for meaningful community involvement and social participation through voluntary organizations and social and leisure activities, and more opportunities for the elderly to be workers, teachers, and leaders in our society. Stricter gun control and stricter restraints on the prescription and distribution of potentially lethal addictive drugs, particularly barbiturates, are other societal changes that would benefit the elderly.

In addition to these broad societal measures, certain specific types of services and therapies are effective in improving the mental health of older adults and in reducing depression and suicide in this group. According to Glasscote, Gudeman, and Miles (1976), three types of services are necessary to promote positive mental health in the aged: (1) supportive services (chore services, telephone assistance, home visits, communal housing, and other services designed to keep the elderly person functioning), (2) clinical services (counseling services, geriatric day care programs, outpatient mental health services), and (3) preventive, supportive, and life-enhancing services (nutrition programs, peer support groups, legal aid, transportation, recreation programs).

Reminiscence and life review therapy has been used effectively with disturbed, depressed older adults (Butler, 1968; Lewis & Butler, 1974; Boylin, Gordon, & Nehrke, 1976; Romaniuk & Romaniuk, 1981). Creative arts therapy--whether through art, music, drama, or dance--is another therapeutic technique which can greatly benefit the elderly (Bright, 1984; Clark & Osgood, 1985; Lerman, 1984; Greenblatt, 1985). Support groups, particularly those for widowed individuals, provide another valuable avenue of treatment for the depressed elderly (Barrett, 1978; Petty, Moeller, & Campbell, 1976; Silverman & Cooperband, 1975). Psychotherapy and group therapy are also beneficial for the elderly (Capuzzi & Gross, 1980; Hartford, 1980; Horton & Linden, 1982). Osgood (1985b, reference 3-034) provides an in-depth discussion of each of these treatment modalities in her book Suicide in the Elderly.

ETHICS AND ELDERLY SUICIDE

The discussion to this point has assumed that prevention of elderly suicide is desirable and is the goal of empirical research of

the phenomenon. There is anything but total agreement regarding
suicide prevention either among the old or generally. Both advocates
and opponents to a right to suicide among the old have put forth their
arguments and concerns. Our society contains groups that attempt to
facilitate or assist those who wish to commit suicide (e.g., the
Hemlock Society, P.O. Box 66218, Los Angeles, CA 90066-0218) and
suicide prevention agencies (in several hundred communities across the
country; a recent list of these agencies may be obtained from the
American Association of Suiciodology, 2459 South Ash Street, Denver, CO
80222). In an attempt to present an issue which becomes of increasing
importance as the number of old and our abilities to prolong life
increase, both sets of arguments surrounding the ethical issues of
elderly suicide will be presented briefly. Before doing so, the reader
who wishes more general writings about the moral, rational, legal,
ethical, and philosophical issues with respect to suicide is directed
to a number of recent books and other works (Basson, 1981; Battin,
1982; Battin & Maris, 1983; Battin & Mayo, 1980; Englehardt &
Malloy, 1982; Litman, 1980; Maris, 1982; Szasz, 1971, reference
3-084) as well as the bibliographies listed in Chapter 2 (especially
McIntosh, 1985, reference 2-007, Chapter 8, pp. 220-244).

Many of those who advocate suicide among the elderly advocate
essentially a "right to die," "a right to self-determination," and
"death with dignity" as the key elements (e.g., Chesser, 1967, Chapter
12; Bromberg & Cassel, 1983, reference 3-076). Doris Portwood (1978,
reference 3-079), in her book Common Sense Suicide: The Final Right,
presents arguments that advocate a right to suicide among elderly
individuals who know it is time for them to die. Portwood discusses
the changes that most often occur with advancing age, particularly the
losses and possibly negative physical, social, and economic changes.
One of the concepts she employs is "balance sheet suicide." That is, a
sane and competent elderly person, "thinking logically [can] . . . set
off the unacceptable or intolerable aspects of his or her life against
the chances for betterment and find the result weighted on the side of
death" (p. 33). That same, or other old persons, may decide however
that the positive aspects outweigh the intolerable and therefore choose
instead life. Portwood's goal is that the opportunity to make this
choice be possible and the mechanism to effect a respectable and
voluntary departure from life be available when "the absence of life
has become more attractive than its presence" (p. 52). She argues that
the quality and not just the quantity of life must be considered.

One author who would undoubtedly agree with Portwood's arguments
is Betty Rollin (1985, reference 3-082), author of the recent book Last
Wish. In this book Rollin describes the plight of her mother, a
76-year-old diagnosed as having ovarian cancer in 1981. Rollin
chronicles the course of her chemotherapy and its negative effects that
finally left the woman wanting to die. She was in great pain and pain
killing medications were ineffective. She had been given six months to
live by doctors and hospice care entailed long waiting lists. She
asked her daughter to help her die. Rollin and her husband contacted
dozens of U.S. doctors, without success, to discover which pills and
how many would allow a painless suicide. Ultimately, an Amsterdam
physician recommended a drug combination. In 1983 Rollin acquired the

drugs, gave them to her mother, and was present when her mother took them while lying in bed.

Another also highly publicized case that has likewise been presented as "rational suicide" is presented in the book Exit House (Roman, 1980) and on film by PBS in the documentary "Choosing Suicide" (broadcast in June 1980). Roman, after learning she had cancer, planned her suicide for fifteen months and at a chosen time at age 60, with many friends and family present she went into a bedroom and took a fatal overdose of seconal. Roman's "fantasy" is for an "Exit House," a place to assist those who wish to die. Others (e.g., Meserve, 1975; Pressey, 1977, reference 3-080) have advocated similar legitimized and institutionalized circumstances to facilitate swift and painless deaths for those elderly who have rationally decided to die.

An additional argument often made for elderly suicide, that very much involves the right to commit suicide, suggests that the death is the choice of the old person and it does not affect or infringe upon the rights of others nor does it harm society (e.g., Alvarez, 1969; Beckwith, 1979; Narveson, 1983; Portwood, 1980, reference 3-079). Lebacqz and Englehardt (1980) justify suicide in terminal illness because in such a situation we cannot fulfill our obligations to others and therefore are not bound by our obligations to them. Invoking the concept of self-determination and the right to autonomy Szasz (1971, reference 3-084) and others (e.g., Bromberg & Cassel, 1983, reference 3-076; Sartorius, 1983) argue that societal intervention with suicide violates one's rights and is unjustified because suicidal ideation does not indicate that a mental illness is present (which may call into question the ability to make rational, considered decisions).

Beyond the issue of the right to commit suicide when an old person has made the rational decision to die, Beckwith (1979) gave six reasons "why [aged] dying persons should be permitted to shorten their painful lives by suicide and why such suicide is beneficial and praiseworthy" (p. 231). These are:

> First and foremost, by timely suicide those dying painfully can end their own suffering immediately. . . . Second, suicide may prevent a degrading or even disgusting death. . . . Third, timely suicide will usually save family and friends the very unpleasant and depressing experience of watching the slow, painful, and degrading death of someone they care for. . . . Fourth, timely suicide by the dying will drastically reduce the often very high cost of dying slowly. . . . funds badly needed for more productive uses. . . . Fifth, dying persons who commit suicide for the above reasons demonstrate the kind of self-control, logical thinking, and considerations for others that most intelligent people respect and admire. . . . Finally, if we legalize and facilitate timely and painless suicide by the dying, we will not only enable them to gain the benefits described above, but will also enable all people to look forward to death with less fear. (pp. 231-232)

In her "Apologia for Suicide," Barrington (1969) argues that a disabled elderly individual in poor health and in need of constant care and attention may feel a burden to the younger person(s) who must provide that care. This situation may be such that the young person is in "bondage" whether willingly or unwillingly. The elderly person may want to "release" the young person but has no real choice but to continue to live on. Barrington argues for the option of voluntary termination of life. Brandt (1975) identified as a morally defensible act cases of suicide that are a response to terminal illness. This may involve release from terrible pain or avoiding great medical expenses which are a burden to the surviving family members.

Finally, Leering, Hilhorst, and Verhoef (1979) suggest that the wish to die in old age may simply be "conscious acceptance of the end of life at life's end" (p. 184). Death is therefore viewed as a natural part of the life cycle.

In addition to the sanctity of life, religious, and other moral arguments, those who feel that suicide should be prevented raise counterarguments to those just presented. One of the most discussed of these arguments suggests that suicide is not or is rarely "rational" (see e.g., Maris, 1982). Some have argued that the suicidal may be mentally ill, most often depressed. Depression may cloud judgment and affect reasoning abilities. A characterization often made regarding the depressed and suicidal is that they have difficulty recognizing or generating alternative solutions to their problems. As Brandt (1975) suggests, they may fail to realize their best solution. To this extent, therefore, suicide may represent not a rational choice weighed against all possible alternatives but only a choice from among few, not necessarily representative, alternatives. Although the terminally ill are most often presented as the example of one who chooses suicide, Siegel and Tuckel (1984-85) note that cancer patients seem to have no elevated suicide risk compared to the general population. The terminally ill who wish suicide may not be as representative of elderly suicides in general as is often suggested.

Maris (1982) points out that there are no guarantees that life will be easy or painless. Indeed, there are no such guarantees about dying either. These elements are part of the unpredictable "human condition" which requires struggle and adaptation. Harsh conditions do not therefore excuse nor legitimize suicide.

It has also been argued that the suicidal are nearly always ambivalent. That is, they wish to die but at the same time they want very much to live. They just may not see any way that that is possible. Ambivalence would argue against the absolute, rational, and clear choice being made. The irreversibility of the choice of suicide is also noted. Would the individual choose suicide at a later time? Might the situation improve, given some time?

Although the advocates of a right to suicide suggest that the suicide affects only the one who dies, it has been argued that we have obligations to others because we are involved in social relationships. Additionally, our act does affect others. The survivors of suicide have often been seen to feel social stigma and perhaps guilt related to the death and the mode of death as suicide may complicate the grief process in a negative fashion (see reviews by Calhoun, Selby, & Selby, 1982; Henley, 1984).

Siegel and Tuckel (1984-85) argue that the legal sanctioning of suicide would undermine societal norms and eliminate clear guidelines in decision making, leading to disorientation and anxiety among those faced with making the decision. Others (e.g., Battin, 1980) have argued that accepting rational suicide may lead to some individuals, and especially the old, being "manipulated" into suicide, perhaps against their will, because they feel obligated (i.e., a duty) to do so in some circumstances. The result then would be to actually lessen free choice. Similarly, Moody (Battin, McKinney, Kastenbaum, & Moody, 1984) worries that the acceptance of suicide as rational "will lead us down the slippery slope" where it is difficult to draw the line at which it is clear when someone is a candidate to commit sanctioned suicide. "Suicide on grounds of old age, not simply during the period of old age" (Moody, 1984, reference 3-078, p. 65) becomes a concern. All disabled elderly under such circumstances could be labeled as living a "meaningless" life. Widespread acceptance of suicide may even encourage suicides that are not rational (e.g., Mayo, 1980).

It is quite clear that this volatile issue has only begun to be presented here. As in any issue with extremely polarized viewpoints and examples that illustrate their points, there is also the middle ground, and the less than clear-cut examples. The ethics of suicide deserve to be addressed. Camus in The Myth of Sysiphus stated that "There is but one philosophical problem: Whether or not to commit suicide." The controversy has recently come to the fore with forces such as life-preserving technology and "how-to" manuals for suicide that have been published in several European countries. The moral dilemma of suicide remains an unresolved issue and the elderly as a group greatly affected are especially involved.

AREAS FOR FUTURE STUDY

At the present time only two books (Miller, 1979, reference 3-027; Osgood, 1985b, reference 3-034) which deal exclusively with the subject of suicide among the elderly have been published. To date this topic has not received the attention it deserves from scholars, researchers, and practitioners, and there are still several areas of study ripe for investigation and inquiry. In this section we will discuss some current problems in the existing state of the art, as well as some of the more fruitful areas of future study.

Problems in Existing U.S. Elderly Suicide Data Bases

Currently we do not know the absolute levels and trends in suicide for older persons, nor do we know the precise nature and characteristics of available data on this population. As John McIntosh (1983) recently pointed out in a symposium on elderly suicide, there are many problems with and inadequacies in suicide data that limit our knowledge of the problem. First, the classification of death as suicide is influenced by the backgrounds and orientations of those who determine the cause of death, as well as by societal taboos and negative sanctions associated with suicide and the circumstances surrounding the death. Secondly, suicide rates are based on both suicide incidence and population figures and inaccuracies in either will affect the computed rates.

In addition to the problems with existing data and suicide rate calculations, there are several limitations in the type of data currently collected, which further limit our ability to describe and explain suicidal behavior in late life. Most importantly, at the present time data are reported in aggregate groups. All those 65+ are grouped together, rendering it impossible to compare various categories of old (e.g., 65–74, 75–84, 85+). Kastenbaum (1985), who recently analyzed suicide data by age in Arizona, discovered a higher rate for the "old–old" as compared to the "young–old." More research on these fast growing populations, particularly the old–old (see e.g., Rosenwaike, 1986; and Suzman & Riley, 1985), are needed (see also McIntosh, 1984, reference 4–059).

Important information such as income, employment status, living conditions, social supports, the presence of physical and/or mental illness, and marital status is not recorded in official mortality data on a national level (since 1979 marital status is once again available in U.S. national data). This type of information is necessary to further our understanding of particularly "at risk" groups of elderly individuals. Similarly, suicide data by age for specific U.S. racial/ethnic minorities are not available in published or unpublished form from the government or any of its agencies. As McIntosh and Santos (1981, reference 4–062) so aptly point out, our existing knowledge of differences in suicidal behaviors for older individuals in different minority groups is very poor although independent research is improving that knowledge base (see McIntosh, 1985). Minority elderly represent a rapidly increasing segment of the U.S. population, one important reason for gaining a better understanding of the mental health needs and problems, including suicidal behavior, of this group.

Cohort Analysis of Suicide Rates

Until fairly recently, researchers have used profile analysis as the major method to study the relationship between suicide and age. This method requires selecting a year or series of years and comparing suicide rates of various age groups, typically grouping data in 5- or 10-year aggregates. Using this method, age-specific suicide rates are calculated and expressed as a number of suicides per 100,000 population within each age group. Once the rates have been calculated, a profile is constructed to allow comparison of rates among various age groups at a particular point or points in time. Profile analysis allows us to determine differences in suicide rates of various age groups at different points in time, however the method does not allow us to determine if, as people age, their risk of suicide increases or decreases. To determine this, one must follow the same birth cohorts over time as they age.

Cohort analysis, which involves following birth cohorts through time as they age, allows us to determine whether changes in suicide patterns are due to aging (maturational effect) or generational differences related to the historical time period of birth (cohort effect). The most recent studies of the relationship between suicide and aging have employed cohort analysis for several countries (Goldney & Katsikitis, 1983, reference 4-029; Lester, 1984, reference 4-047; Murphy & Wetzel, 1980, reference 4-069; Pollinger-Haas & Hendin, 1983, reference 3-042; Reed, Camus, & Last, 1985, reference 4-080; Solomon & Hellon, 1980, reference 4-094; Solomon & Murphy, 1984, reference 4-095). These studies have reached similar conclusions: suicide rates appear to be increasing in younger age groups for each successive birth cohort since 1950, and within each cohort suicide rates have increased directly with age. One of the limitations of this research thus far is that the birth cohorts in which these increased rates at successive ages have been observed have not yet reached old age. It is not yet apparent whether this continued increase with age will continue as these birth cohorts age. Pollinger-Haas and Hendin (1983, reference 3-042) suggest that the rate increases will continue due to the increased number of individuals in these cohorts who will experience increased stress associated with such large numbers in population. Ahlburg and Schapiro (1984, reference 4-003) agree with Pollinger-Haas and Hendin regarding cohort size and add the effects such numbers in the population will have on work force participation. Holinger and Offer's (1982, reference 4-033) comments, however, disagree with those of Pollinger-Haas and Hendin as well as Ahlburg and Shapiro. Holinger and Offer suggest that the increasing number of old among the currently large young cohorts may lead to increased attention and benefits rather than increased stress and competitiveness. Such outcomes of large cohort size may work to lessen rather than increase the likelihood of suicide when these cohorts become old. To further our understanding of maturational versus cohort effects on suicidal behavior, it is necessary to follow current cohorts as they age, particularly the "baby boomers" who are currently beginning to enter their 40s, and perform cohort analyses in the future.

Indirect Life-Threatening Behavior

Few studies have examined the nature and extent of what has been variously referred to as "hidden suicide" (Meerloo, 1968, reference 3-025), or "indirect life-threatening behavior" (Nelson & Farberow, 1980, reference 4-072). Indirect life-threatening behavior (ILTB) is defined as repetitive acts by individuals directed toward themselves which result in physical harm or tissue damage and which could bring about a premature end of life (for a more general consideration of a variety of indirect self-destructive behavior, see Farberow, 1980). Examples of ILTB include: refusing to eat or drink, refusing medications, or refusing to follow specified medical regimens. Some of the investigations which have been conducted reveal a fairly high incidence of ILTB among patients in long-term care facilities that have been studied (Mishara & Kastenbaum, 1973, reference 4-067; Nelson, 1977, reference 4-070; Nelson & Farberow, 1980, reference 4-072). One of these studies (Nelson & Farberow, 1980) further suggests that some of the same characteristics which are related to overt suicide are also factors in ILTB. However, our knowledge of this behavior among the elderly is very limited. Currently we do not know how many older adults in the community and in institutions engage in such behavior. Nor do we know which types of older adults are most likely to choose these less overt forms of self-destructive behavior and how they compare to older adults who commit overt suicide. Studies of the extent and nature of this type of suicidal behavior among the old are badly needed.

Suicide in the Institutionalized Elderly

There are approximately 23,000 long-term care facilities serving 5% of the elderly in this country at any one time. Very little research on suicide among elderly residents of long-term care facilities has been conducted. Few studies have examined the extent and nature of overt suicide or attempted suicide in long-term care institutions. One study conducted on the geriatric ward of a Veterans Administration medical center (Wolff, 1970a, reference 4-110) suggests that overt suicide does occur in long-term care facilities.

We currently do not know how many residents of long-term care facilities commit overt suicide, attempt suicide, or engage in ILTB. We also have very little knowledge of how these behaviors vary by sex, race, and age. Do men engage in overt suicide more frequently than women in such institutional settings? Do whites engage in ILTB more frequently than nonwhites? What is the profile of the most "at risk" institutionalized resident and how does it differ from that for the elderly as a whole? These and other questions regarding the nature of suicide and ILTB among residents of long-term care facilities cannot satisfactorily be answered at the present time. We also do not currently know whether older individuals living in long-term care institutions commit suicide, attempt suicide, or engage in ILTB more than older individuals in the general population. These and other important questions offer a fruitful area for future research. Dr. Nancy Osgood is presently conducting a study of the extent and nature of suicide in long-term care facilities and the effect of facility and staff characteristics--such as size, provisions for privacy, staff to patient ratio--on such behavior. Results of this study should be published/available in 1987 from Aspen Systems Corporation.

Cross-Cultural Comparisons

The World Health Organization (WHO) collects and publishes suicide statistics by age groups for selected countries. A few researchers have used these statistics to analyze cross-cultural differences in late life suicide and have offered various macro-cultural explanations for such differences (Altergott, 1983; Atchley, 1980, reference 4-004; Berdes, 1978, reference 3-006; Kruijt, 1977, reference 4-042).

By conducting a national-level analysis, Atchley (1980, reference 3-004) could show that age interacts with socio-cultural context in producing suicide and that several distinct patterns exist. In many countries, suicide was strongly correlated with age (England & Wales,

Germany, Austria, Switzerland, Hungary) while it was less strongly, but still positively, correlated with age in other countries (Canada, Finland, Australia for women). Similar cross-cultural analyses of data have produced more than one suicide pattern by age (see e.g., Jedlicka, 1978, reference 4-035; and Ruzicka, 1976, reference 4-082).

Atchley also examined the impact of several structural conditions, such as degree of urbanization and gross national product of different countries. Age patterns in suicide for women were found highly related to economic conditions. As economic conditions improve, the strong positive correlation between age and suicide decreases in strength.

In her recent analysis of cross-cultural differences in suicide rates for the old in 11 countries, Altergott (1983) found great cross-national variation in the age pattern of suicide, refuting the notion that there is anything biologically or chronologically given about the increase in suicide with age. Altergott suggests, rather, that her findings lead to questions concerning variable structural and cultural conditions that differentially impact the age and gender groups in different countries. At the present time we do not have answers to such questions. While studies have been done by the WHO on the mental and physical health of the aged in many countries, few analyses on the relationship between individual condition and risk of suicide have been conducted. This area of inquiry offers several opportunities for future research.

Suicide Prevention and Postvention

Suicide prevention and promotion of positive mental health among our aged should be a major goal in this and other countries. Unfortunately, the limitations in our existing data and knowledge base, some of which have just been discussed, seriously hamper our efforts at suicide prevention. At the present time we have limited information regarding the particular effects of various forms of intervention and therapy on suicide prevention and how such techniques differentially impact different types of older persons. Such information is needed if we are to reduce the suicide rate among the old. The psychological autopsy (see e.g., Weisman & Kastenbaum, 1968), which involves finding out "after the fact" about the personal relationships, previous suicidal attempts and/or threats, and clues to suicidal behavior given by the victim, is intended to determine the extent to which the individual played a role in their death. Such a technique may increase our knowledge and aid ultimately in suicide prevention. Researchers and clinicians could pursue this form of intensive research.

A fairly new area of focus is on the survivors who remain after the suicide has been completed (reviews of this literature may be found in Calhoun et al., 1982, and Henley, 1984). Postvention is the term which is being used to refer to dealing with the socio-emotional effects on the loved ones left behind. John McIntosh, Karen Dunne-Maxim, Edward Dunne, and Carol Billow-Borowka are currently editing a book on survivors of suicide which should increase our knowledge of this group (should be available in 1987 from W. W. Norton). Norman Farberow, Dolores Gallagher, and colleagues are also currently conducting research on survivors, including survivors of elderly suicide. Preliminary results of their work were reported at the International Meetings in Gerontology in July 1985. David Shaffer and colleagues at Columbia University have also received a large federal grant to study survivors of suicide. Results of their study should be available in 1987 or 1988. The only research findings thus far published which focus attention on survivors of elderly suicide was the study of suicides in Singapore by Chia (1979, reference 4-016). This study's results, however, share a methodological difficulty common to present studies of survivors of suicide. No comparison/control group of survivors of other causes of death or of suicide survivors of other ages were included in the design. Without such comparison groups, the results are open to alternative explanations and are not fully interpretable or useful. Methodologically sound research in this area regarding survivors of all ages is sorely needed.

REFERENCES NOT INCLUDED IN ANNOTATIONS

Altergott, K. (1983, November 19). Qualities of daily life and suicide in old age: A comparative perspective. Paper presented at the annual meeting of the Gerontological Society of America, San Francisco.

Alvarez, W. C. (1969, October). Is suicide by an old, dying person a sin and a crime? [Editorial]. Geriatrics, 24(10), 77-78.

American Association of Retired Persons. (1980). Rank order of retirement problems. Unpublished report, Andrus Gerontology Center, University of Southern California, Los Angeles, CA.

Andress, V. R., & Corey, D. M. (1978). Survivor-victims: Who discovers or witnesses suicide? Psychological Reports, 42, 759-764.

Atchley, R. C. (1976). The sociology of retirement. New York: Wiley.

Barrett, C. J. (1978). Effectiveness of widows' groups in facilitating change. Journal of Consulting and Clinical Psychology, 46, 20-31.

Barrington, M. R. (1969). Apologia for suicide. In A. B. Downing (Ed.) Euthanasia and the right to die (pp. 152-172). London: Peter Owen.

Basson, M. D. (Ed.). (1981). Rational suicide. Progress in Clinical and Biological Research, 50, 179-212.

Battin, M. P. (1980). Manipulated suicide. Bioethics Quarterly, 2, 123-134.

Battin, M. P. (1982). Ethical issues in suicide. Englewood Cliffs, NJ: Prentice-Hall.

Battin, M. P., & Maris, R. W. (Eds.). (1983). Suicide and ethics (special issue of Suicide and Life-Threatening Behavior, 13(4)).

New York: Human Sciences Press.

Battin, M. P., & Mayo, D. J. (Eds.). (1980). Suicide: The
philosophical issues. New York: St. Martin's Press.

Battin, M. P., McKinney, D., Kastenbaum, R., & Moody, H. R. (1984).
Suicide: A solution to the problem of old age. In C. R. Pfeffer &
J. Richman (Eds.), Proceedings of the 15th annual meeting of the
American Association of Suicidology (April 1982, New York City)
(pp. 78–81). Denver, CO: American Association of Suicidology.
[Abstract]

Beck, A. T. (1967). Depression: Causes and treatment.   Philadelphia:
University of Pennsylvania Press.

Beckwith, B. P. (1979).   On the right to suicide by the   dying.
Dissent, 26, 231–233.

Berardo, F. M. (1967).   Social adaptation to widowhood among a
rural–urban aged population (Washington Agricultural Experiment
Station Bulletin No. 689). Pullman: Washington State University.

Berardo, F. M. (1968). Widowhood status in the U.S.: Perspectives on
a neglected aspect of the family life cycle. Family Coordinator,
17, 191–203.

Berardo, F. M. (1970). Survivorship and social isolation: The case of
the aged widower. Family Coordinator, 19, 11 25.

Bidder, T. G. (1981). Electroconvulsive therapy in the medically ill
patient. Psychiatric Clinics of North America, 4, 391–406.

Birren, J. E., & Sloane, R. B. (Eds.). (1980).   Handbook of mental
health and aging. Englewood Cliffs, NJ: Prentice-Hall.

Blau, Z. S. (1956).   Changes in status and age identification.
American Sociological Review, 21, 198–203.

Blazer, D. (1982). Depression in late life. St. Louis, MO: Mosby.

Borson, S., & Veith, R. C. (1985). Pharmacological interventions.   In
N. J. Osgood, Suicide in the elderly: A practitioner's guide to
diagnosis and mental health interventions (pp. 116–130). Rockville,
MD: Aspen Systems.

Boylin, W., Gordon, S. K., & Nehrke, M. R. (1976). Reminiscing and ego
integrity in institutionalized elderly males.   Gerontologist, 16,
118–124.

Brandt, R. B. (1975). The morality and rationality of suicide.   In
S. Perlin (Ed.), A handbook for the study of suicide (pp. 61–76).
New York: Oxford University Press.

Breed, W. (1963). Occupational mobility and suicide among white males.

American Sociological Review, 28, 179–188.

Bright, R. (1984). _Music in geriatric care_ (2nd ed.).   Sherman Oaks, CA: Alfred Publishing.

Butler, R. N. (1968).   The life review: An interpretation of reminiscence in the aged. In B. L. Neugarten (Ed.), _Middle age and aging_ (pp. 486–496). Chicago: University of Chicago Press.

Butler, R. N. (1975). _Why survive? Being old in America_.   New York: Harper & Row.

Calhoun, L. G., Selby, J. W., & Selby, L. E. (1982).   The psychological aftermath of suicide: An analysis of current evidence.   _Clinical Psychology Review_, 2, 409–420.

Capuzzi, D., & Gross, D. (1980). Group work with the elderly: An overview for counselors.   _Personnel and Guidance Journal_, 58, 206–211.

Carroll, B. J., Feinburg, M., Greden, J. F., Tarika, J., Albala, A. A., Haskett, R. F., James, N. M., Kronfol, Z., Lohr, N., Steiner, M., de Vigne, J. P., & Young, E. (1981). A specific laboratory test for the diagnosis of melancholia: Standardization, validation, and clinical utility. _Archives of General Psychiatry_, 30, 15–22.

Cassano, G. B., Maggini, C., & Akiskai, H. S. (1983).   Short-term, subchronic, and chronic sequalae of affective disorders. _Psychiatric Clinics of North America_, 6, 55–68.

Cath, S. H. (1965). Discussion notes. In M. A. Berezin & S. H. Cath (Eds.), _Geriatric psychiatry: Grief, loss and emotional disorder in the aging process_ (pp. 128–129). New York: International Universities Press.

Centers for Disease Control. (1985, June 21). Suicide––United States, 1970–1980. _Morbidity and Mortality Weekly Report_, 34(24), 353–357.

Chaisson, G. M. (1981). Depression in the elderly. In S. Anderson & E. E. Bahwens (Eds.), _Chronic health problems: Concepts and application_ (pp. 262–273). St. Louis, MO: Mosby.

Chesser, E. (1967). _Living with suicide_. London: Hutchinson.

Clark, P. A., & Osgood, N. J. (1985). _Seniors on stage: The impact of applied theatre techniques on the elderly_. New York: Praeger.

Coble, P. A., Kupfer, D. J., & Shaw, D. H. (1981). Distribution of REM latency in depression. _Biological Psychology_, 16, 453–456.

Cowgill, D. O.,   & Holmes, L. D. (Eds.). (1972).   _Aging   and modernization_. New York: Appleton–Century–Crofts.

Englehardt, H. T., Jr., & Malloy, M. (1982).   Suicide and assisting suicide: A critique of legal sanctions. Southwestern Law Journal, 36, 1003-1037.

Erikson, E. H. (1963). Childhood and society (2nd rev. ed.). New York: Norton.

Farber, M. L. (1968). Theory of suicide. New York: Funk & Wagnalls.

Farberow, N. L. (Ed.). (1980). The many faces of suicide: Indirect self-destructive behavior. New York: McGraw-Hill.

Friedel, R. O. (1982). The diagnosis and management of depression in the elderly patient. In C. Eisdorfer & W. E. Fann (Eds.), Treatment of psychopathology in the aging (pp. 210-217). New York: Springer.

Gaitz, C. M., & Varner, R. V. (1980). Adjustment disorders of late life: Stress disorders. In E. Busse & D. Glazer (Eds.), Handbook of geriatric psychiatry (pp. 381-389). New York: Van Nostrand Reinhold.

Gerner, R. H. (1979). Depression in the elderly. In O. J. Kaplan (Ed.), Psychopathology of aging (pp. 97-148). New York: Academic Press.

Giddens, A. (Ed.). (1971). The sociology of suicide. London: Frank Cass & Co.

Glamser, F. D., & DeJong, G. F. (1975). The efficacy of preretirement programs for industrial workers. Journal of Gerontology, 30, 595-599.

Glasscote, R., Gudeman, J. E., & Miles, C. D. (1976). Creative mental health services for the elderly. Washington, D.C.: American Psychiatric Association.

Greenblatt, F. S. (1985). Drama with the elderly: Acting at eighty. Springfield, IL: Thomas.

Gubrium, J. F. (1974). Marital desolation and the evaluation of everyday life in old age. Journal of Marriage and the Family, 36, 107-113.

Gurland, B. J., & Cross, P. S. (1983). Suicide among the elderly. In M. K. Aronson, R. Bennett, & B. J. Gurland (Eds.), The acting-out elderly (pp. 55-65). New York: Haworth Press.

Hamilton, M. (1960). A rating scale for depression. Journal of Neurology, Neurosurgery, and Psychiatry, 23, 56-62.

Hartford, M. E. (1980). The use of group methods for work with the aged. In J. E. Birren & R. Sloane (Eds.), Handbook of mental health and aging (pp. 806-826). Englewood Cliffs, NJ: Prentice-Hall.

Hatton, C. L., Valente, S. M., & Rink, A. (Eds.). (1977). Suicide:

Assessment and intervention. New York: Appleton–Century–Crofts.

Henley, S. H. A. (1984, Summer). Bereavement following suicide: A review of the literature. *Current Psychological Research and Reviews*, 3(2), 53–61.

Henry, A., & Short, J. F. (1954). *Suicide and homicide*. Glencoe, IL: Free Press.

Horton, A. M., & Linden, M. E. (1982). Geriatric group psychotherapy. In A. Horton (Ed.), *Mental health interventions for the aging* (pp. 51–68). New York: Praeger.

Kastenbaum, R. (1972). While the old man dies: Our conflicting attitudes. In B. Schoenberg, A. C. Carr, D. Peretz, & A. H. Kutscher (Eds.), *Psychosocial aspects of terminal care* (pp. 116–125). New York: Columbia University Press.

Kastenbaum, R. (1985, July). *"Why go on?" Suicidal thoughts and actions in later life*. Paper presented at the 13th meeting of the International Congress on Gerontology, New York.

Kendell, R. E. (1981). The present status of electroconvulsive treatment. *British Journal of Psychiatry*, 139, 265–283.

Lebacqz, K., & Englehardt, H. T. (1980). Suicide and covenant. In M. P. Battin & D. J. Mayo (Eds.), *Suicide: The philosophical issues* (pp. 84–89). New York: St. Martin's Press.

Leering, C., Hilhorst, H. W. A., & Verhoef, M. J. (1979). Reflections on the wish to die at life's end. In H. Orimo, K. Shimada, M. Iriki, & D. Maeda (Eds.), *Recent advances in gerontology* (pp. 183–184). Amsterdam: Excerpta Medica.

Lehr, U. (1981). Stereotypes of aging and age norms. In D. Danon, N. W. Shock, & N. Maroes (Eds.), *Proceedings of the World Conference of Institute de la Vie, Volume 3, Aging: A challenge to science and society* (pp. 101–112). Oxford, England: Oxford University Press.

Lerman, L. (1984). *Teaching dance to senior adults*. Springfield, IL: Thomas.

Lewis, M. L., & Butler, R. N. (1974). Life–review therapy: Putting memories to work in individual and group psychotherapy. *Geriatrics*, 29(11), 165–173.

Litman, R. E. (1980). Psycholegal aspects of suicide. In W. J. Curran, A. L. McGarry, & C. S. Petty (Eds.), *Modern legal medicine: Psychiatry and forensic science* (pp. 841–853). Philadelphis: Davis.

Litman, R., Curphey, T., Shneidman, E., Farberow, N., & Tabachnick, N. (1963). Investigations of equivocal suicide. *Journal of the American Medical Association*, 184, 924–929.

Loether, H. J. (1975). Problems of aging: Sociological and social psychological perspectives (2nd ed.). Belmont, CA: Dickerson Publishing.

Loosen, P. T., & Prange, A. J., Jr. (1982). Serum thyrotropin response to thyrotropin-releasing hormones in psychiatric patients: A review. American Journal of Psychiatry, 139, 405-416.

Malloy, F. W., Small, I. F., Miller, M. J., Milstein, V., & Stout, J. R. (1982). Changes in neuropsychological test performance after electroconvulsive therapy. Biological Psychiatry, 17, 61-67.

Maris, R. W. (1969). Social forces in urban suicide. Homewood, IL: Dorsey.

Maris, R. W. (1982). Rational suicide: An impoverished self-transformation. Suicide and Life-Threatening Behavior, 12, 4-16.

Mayo, D. J. (1980). Irrational suicide. In M. P. Battin & D. J. Mayo (Eds.), Suicide: The philosophical issues (pp. 133-137). New York: St. Martin's Press.

McIntosh, J. L. (1983, November 19). Official U.S. elderly suicide data bases: Levels, availability, omissions. Paper presented at the annual meeting of the Gerontological Society of America, San Francisco.

McIntosh, J. L. (1984a). Suicide among children, adolescents, and students, 1980-1984: A comprehensive bibliography. Monticello, IL: Vance Bibliographies, Public Administration Series Bibliography P-1586.

McIntosh, J. L. (1985, November 24). Suicide among minority elderly. Paper presented at the annual meeting of the Gerontological Society of America, New Orleans, LA.

McIntosh, J. L., Hubbard, R. W., & Santos, J. F. (1980, November 24). Suicide among nonwhite elderly: 1960-1977. Paper presented at the annual meeting of the Gerontological Society of America, San Diego, CA.

McIntosh, J. L., & Jewell, B. L. (1986). Sex difference trends in completed suicide. Suicide and Life-Threatening Behavior, 16, 16-27.

Meier-Ruge, W. (1975). From our laboratories. Triangle, 14, 71-72.

Melville, M. L., & Blazer, D. G. (1985). Depression in the elderly: Etiology and assessment. In N. J. Osgood, Suicide in the elderly: A practitioner's guide to diagnosis and mental health intervention (pp. 14-38). Rockville, MD: Aspen Systems.

Menninger, K. (1938). Man against himself. New York: Harcourt, Brace & World.

Meserve, H. C. (1975). Getting out of it. Journal of Religion and Health, 14, 3-6.

Miller, M. (1976). Suicide among older men (Doctoral dissertation, University of Michigan, 1976). Dissertation Abstracts International, 37, 3156B. (University Microfilms 76-27,546)

Mizruchi, E. H. (1964). Success and opportunity. Glencoe, IL: Free Press.

Mizruchi, E. H. (1982). Abeyance process and time: An exploratory approach to age and social structure. In E. Mizruchi, B. Glassner, & T. Pastorello (Eds.), Time and aging (pp. 112-128). Bayside, NY: General Hall, Inc.

Morgan, H. G. (1979). Death wishes? The understanding and management of deliberate self-harm. New York: Wiley.

Narveson, J. (1983). Self-ownership and the ethics of suicide. In M. P. Battin & R. W. Maris (Eds.), Suicide and ethics (pp. 240-253). New York: Human Sciences Press.

Neugarten, B. L. (Ed.). (1968a). Middle age and aging.   Chicago: University of Chicago Press.

Neugarten, B. L. (1968b). The awareness of middle age. In B. L. Neugarten (Ed.), Middle age and aging (pp. 93-98). Chicago: University of Chicago Press.

Oliven, J. F. (1951). The suicidal risk: Its diagnosis and evaluation. New England Journal of Medicine, 245, 488-494.

Palmore, E. (1982). Preparation for retirement: The impact of preretirement programs on retirement and leisure. In N. J. Osgood (Ed.), Life after work: Retirement, leisure, recreation, and the elderly (pp. 330-341). New York: Praeger.

Palmore, E., & Manton, K. (1974). Modernization and status of the aged: International correlations. Journal of Gerontology, 29, 205-210.

Petty, B. J., Moeller, T. P., & Campbell, R. Z. (1976). Support groups for elderly persons in the community. Gerontologist, 16, 522-528.

Pfeiffer, E. (1977). Psychopathology and social pathology. In J. E. Birren & K. W. Schaie (Eds.), Handbook of the psychology of aging (pp. 650-671). New York: Van Nostrand Reinhold.

Powell, E. H. (1970). The design of discord. New York: Oxford University Press.

Quinney, R. (1965). Suicide, homicide and economic development. Social Forces, 43, 401-406.

Robins, A. H. (1976). Depression in patients with Parkinsonism. British Journal of Psychiatry, 128, 141-145.

Roman, J. (1980). Exit house: Choosing suicide as an alternative. New York: Seaview Books.

Romaniuk, M., & Romaniuk, J. (1981). Looking back: An analysis of reminiscence functions and triggers. Experimental Aging Research, 7, 477-489.

Rosenwaike, I. (1986). The extreme aged in America: A portrait of an expanding population. Westport, CT: Greenwood Press.

Rosow, I. (1967). Social integration of the aged. New York: Free Press.

Rosow, I. (1973). The social context of the aging self. Gerontologist, 12, 82-87.

Salzman, C., & Shader, R. (1979). Clinical evaluation of depression in the elderly. In A. Raskin & L. Jarvik (Eds.), Psychiatric symptoms and cognitive loss in the elderly (pp. 39-57). New York: Hemisphere.

Sartorius, R. (1983). Coercive suicide prevention: A libertarian perspective. In M. P. Battin & R. W. Maris (Eds.), Suicide and ethics (pp. 293-303). New York: Human Sciences Press.

Schulz, R. (1976). Effects of control and predictability on the physical and psychological well-being of the institutionalized aged. Journal of Personality and Social Psychology, 33, 563-573.

Seligman, M. E. P. (1975). Helplessness. San Francisco: Freeman.

Seligman, M. E. P. (1976). Learned helplessness and depression in animals and men. In J. T. Spence, R. C. Carsen, & J. W. Thibaut (Eds.), Behavioral approaches to therapy (pp. 111-126). Morristown, NJ: General Learning Press.

Shneidman, E. S. (1969). Prologue: Fifty-eight years. In E. S. Shneidman (Ed.), On the nature of suicide (pp. 1-30). San Francisco: Jossey Bass.

Siegal, K., & Tuckel, P. (1984-85). Rational suicide and the terminally ill cancer patient. Omega, 15, 263-269.

Silverman, P. S., & Cooperband, A. (1975). On widowhood mutual help and the elderly widow. Journal of Geriatric Psychiatry, 8, 9-27.

Spiker, D. G., Coble, P., Cofsky, J., Foster, F. G., & Kupfer, D. J. (1978). EEG sleep and severity of depression. Biological Psychiatry, 13, 485-488.

Suzman, R., & Riley, M. W. (Eds.). (1985, Spring). Special issue: The oldest old. *Milbank Memorial Fund Quarterly: Health and Society*, 63(Whole No. 2).

Tedrick, T. (1982). Leisure competency: A goal for aging Americans in the 1980s. In N. J. Osgood (Ed.), *Life after work: Retirement, leisure, recreation, and the elderly* (pp. 315–318). New York: Praeger.

Townsend, P. (1968). Isolation, desolation, and loneliness. In E. Shanas, P. Townsend, D. Wedderbury, H. Frus, P. Milkof, & G. Stehower (Eds.), *Old people in three industrial societies* (pp. 258–287). New York: Atherton Press.

Troll, L. E., Israel, J., & Israel, K. (1977). *Looking ahead: A woman's guide to the problems and joys of growing older*. Englewood Cliffs, NJ: Prentice–Hall.

Tuckman, J. (1970). Suicide and the suicide prevention center. In K. Wolff (Ed.), *Patterns of self-destruction: Depression and suicide* (pp. 18–28). Springfield, IL: Thomas.

Weisman, A. D., & Kastenbaum, R. (1968). *The psychological autopsy: A study of the terminal phase of life*. New York: Behavioral Publications. (Community Mental Health Journal Monograph No. 4)

Wekstein, L. (1979). *Handbook of suicidology: Principles, problems, and practice*. New York: Brunner/Mazel.

Williams, R. M., Jr. (1970). *American society*. New York: Knopf.

Wilson, L. G. (1976). Viral encephalopathy mimicking functional psychosis. *American Journal of Psychiatry*, 133, 165–170.

Wolff, K. (1970). *The emotional rehabilitation of the geriatric patient*. Springfield, IL: Thomas.

Zung, W. K. (1965). A self-rating depression scale. *Archives of General Psychiatry*, 12, 63–70.

2
BIBLIOGRAPHIC SOURCES
ON ELDERLY SUICIDE

Few bibliographies on elderly suicide exist. This chapter presents published bibliographic sources on elderly suicide as well as more general bibliographies on suicide. For the reader who wishes to extend the citations of this book, abstract and index sources in which references on elderly suicide appear are also listed. For more exhaustive and extensive listings of index and abstract sources with respect to suicide see McIntosh (1985, reference 2-007) or Lester, Sell, and Sell (1980, reference 2-005).

Research and review works on suicide and suicide among the elderly may appear in journals and books from a large number of fields of study because of the multidisciplinary nature of both gerontology and suicidology. The most likely sources, however, are journals in psychology, psychiatry, sociology, and thanatology. There are four journals in particular which publish writings on suicide and death and dying that are especially likely to yield articles of interest. These four are: Crisis: International Journal of Suicide- and Crisis-Studies, Essence: Issues in the Study of Ageing, Dying, and Death, Omega: Journal of Death and Dying, and Suicide and Life-Threatening Behavior.

BIBLIOGRAPHIES ON ELDERLY SUICIDE

2-001 McIntosh, John L. (1981b). Suicide among the elderly: A comprehensive bibliography. Monticello, IL: Vance Bibliographies, Public Administration Series Bibliography No. P-686.

This 37 page non-annotated bibliography includes references through 1979 and early 1980 on elderly suicide as well as age in general. The citations most often include the source of abstracts for the references included. Non-English articles are also included.

2-002 McIntosh, John L. (1984b). Suicide among the elderly, 1980-1984: A comprehensive bibliography. Monticello, IL: Vance Bibliographies, Public Administraction Series Bibliography No. P-1584.

This 10 page non-annotated bibliography supplements and updates McIntosh, 1981b, reference 2-001 above. The information included in the above reference appears also in this supplement and a separate set of listings on middle age suicide references is also included.

2-003   Miller, Marv. (1979). A review of the research on geriatric suicide. Death Education, 3, 282-296. (Adapted from Miller, Marv. (1979). Suicide after sixty: The final alternative. New York: Springer.)

In addition to reviewing the literature on elderly suicide, Miller includes a table which summarizes research reports on the topic. These quite brief annotations and tabular notations are informative but much less detailed than the annotations found in the present work. This same table with its abstracts is included in an appendix to the 1979 book noted in this citation. The 19 abstracted articles were published from 1951 to 1977.

GENERAL BIBLIOGRAPHIC SOURCES ON SUICIDE

2-004   Farberow, Norman L. (1972). Bibliography on suicide and suicide prevention: 1897-1957, 1958-1970. Washington, D.C.: United States Government Printing Office, DHEW Publication No. (HSM) 72-9080 (Revision of PHS Publication No. 1970, originally published, 1969). SuDoc Number: HE 20.2417: Su3

This is the most comprehensive bibliography on suicide to 1970. Subject and author indexes are included and the work is divided into sections by the groupings of references published from 1897 to 1957 and those appearing from 1958 to 1970.

2-005   Lester, David, Sell, Betty H., & Sell, Kenneth D. (1980). Suicide: A guide to information sources. Detroit: Gale Research Company.

This bibliographic source gives great attention to index, abstract, and general sources of information about suicide but includes few specific references on particular topics. It is an excellent source for the individual wishing to perform an exhaustive search for materials in little known reference locations.

2-006   Gallagher, Dolores, & Kronauer, Margaret L. (1981). Depression in the elderly: A selected bibliography. Los Angeles: Ethel Percy Andrus Gerontology Center, University of Southern California (Technical Bibliographies on Aging Series).

This non-annotated bibliography includes a section on suicide (pp. 48-57) that is grouped into references on epidemiology, evaluation of risk factors, and interventions.

2-007 McIntosh, John L. (1985). <u>Research on suicide: A bibliography</u>.
       Westport, CT: Greenwood Press.

       This over 2300-citation categorized bibliography presents mostly
       non-annotated references on a comprehensive array of subtopics
       for suicide.   A section on age as well as the elderly
       (pp. 79-83) are included. Subject and author indexes are also
       included. While not intended to be exhaustive, this is the most
       comprehensive bibliography from a topical viewpoint since
       Farberow (1972, reference 2-004) which covered the literature to
       1970. Most of the references in this bibliography are since
       1970.

2-008 Poteet, G. Howard, & Santora, Joseph C. (1978).   <u>Death and</u>
       <u>dying: A bibliography, 1950-1974</u>. <u>Supplement Volume 1,</u>
       <u>Suicide</u>. Troy, NY: Whitson Publishing.

       This topically arranged bibliography presents a mix of
       professional and popular press references on a large number of
       subtopics about suicide. An author index is included.

2-009 Prentice, Ann E. (1974). <u>Suicide: A selective bibliography of</u>
       <u>over 2,200 items</u>. Metuchen, NJ: Scarecrow Press.

       This bibliography is arranged by type of works (books, journal
       articles, dissertations, popular press, etc.).   Subject and
       author indexes are included.

INDEX AND ABSTRACT SOURCES FOR REFERENCES ON ELDERLY SUICIDE

2-010 <u>Current Contents, Social and Behavioral Sciences</u> (published
       weekly)

2-011 <u>Current Literature on Aging</u> (published quarterly by the National
       Council on Aging)

2-012 <u>Dissertation Abstracts International</u> (published monthly) [Note:
       Each year in the <u>Journal of Gerontology</u> there appears an article
       that lists the doctoral dissertations in gerontology. These
       dissertations are listed by topics and when appropriate the
       heading of "Suicide" is included.]

2-013 <u>Excerpta Medica</u>, Section 20:   Geriatrics, Section 32:
       Psychiatry

2-014 <u>Gerontological Abstracts</u>

2-015 <u>Index Medicus</u> (published monthly)

2-016 <u>Psychological Abstracts</u> (published monthly)

2-017 <u>Social Sciences Citation Index</u> (published quarterly)

2-018 <u>Sociological Abstracts</u> (published bimonthly)

3
OVERVIEW AND OTHER NON-EMPIRICAL WORKS: ANNOTATIONS

OVERVIEW WORKS

3-001 Barraclough, B. M. (1971). Suicide in the elderly. In
D. W. K. Kay & Alexander Walk (Eds.), Recent developments in
psychogeriatrics (pp. 87–97). Ashford, Kent: Headley Brothers
Limited.

The author summarizes the findings of Sainsbury (1963, reference
4–085, and 1968, reference 4–086) on elderly suicide with
respect to the methodology of the research, the diagnosis of
mental illness and suicide, the symptoms displayed, the duration
of illnesses, recent medical care received by the suicides,
physical illness and suicide, living alone, and anniversaries
and suicide. Barraclough suggests that the treatment of
depressive older persons may lessen suicidal ideation, that the
elderly often do not know of the availability of suicide
prevention services, and that the old in need of help may need
it brought to them because they do not appreciate their own
need. The author suggests that psychiatrists work more closely
with the family members of the chronically depressed and that
careful follow-up of the depressed may help to lessen suicidal
risk. Barraclough suggests the inclusion of more information on
death certificates and in coroners' inquest notes. He concludes
that much research needs to be done and among the particular
needs is the careful, planned evaluation of prevention measures.

3-002 Batchelor, I. R. C. (1955). Management and prognosis of
suicidal attempts in old age. Geriatrics, 10, 291–293.

Batchelor begins this overview of the management and prognosis
of elderly suicide with a case of a suicide attempt of a
90-year-old widower. The author suggests that at least 80% of
the suicidal elderly are "suffering from depressions" and "all
suicidal old people . . . are depressed" (p. 291). Because the
old rarely make suicidal gestures, the act must be taken
seriously and any attempt requires a comprehensive review of the
psychosocial environment of the old person. The presence of
physical or mental illness should be determined and the home
situation should be investigated and if involved in the suicide

attempt should be corrected before the person's return to it.
Follow-up results of attempters indicate that the old are at
greater risk for subsequent suicide than are younger
individuals. Finally, Batchelor notes the rigidity (i.e.,
sameness in attempts) for the elderly as a factor that should
facilitate prevention.

3-003 Batchelor, I. R. C. (1957). Suicide in old age. In
Edwin S. Shneidman & Norman L. Farberow (Eds.), Clues to suicide
(pp. 143-151). New York: McGraw-Hill.

This article offers a good review of the early research findings
on elderly suicide. The findings of O'Neal et al. (1956,
reference 4-073) and Batchelor and Napier (1953, reference
4-008) are the primary results that are reviewed. Batchelor
notes that "It is probable that in old age attempted suicides
and suicides fall into clinical groups which, if not identical,
are very closely allied. In old age, a suicidal attempt is
rarely a gesture or threat; it is usually a suicide which has
failed for reasons other than the seriousness and determination
of the actor" (p. 144). The author suggests that the mental
illness that the suicidal old person is suffering at the time is
the most important factor. The loss of others is an important
factor as well, and it is suggested that at least one-fourth of
all suicidal attempts among the young and old are attempts to
rejoin a dead person. Prevention methods suggested include the
continued integration of the old in work, family, and community
groups, and early treatment of mental illness.

3-004 Bennett, A. E. (1967). Recognizing the potential suicide.
Geriatrics, 22, 175-181.

One of the first statements Bennett makes is that "If suicidal
patients could be recognized early and handled properly, maybe
50% of them could be saved" (p. 175). The author points out the
high proportion of elderly who see their physician shortly
before their suicide and the opportunity this provides for
recognition and prevention. Danger signals or clues to suicide
are briefly discussed. It is concluded that (1) it is the
responsibility of a physician to prevent suicide, (2) that
follow-up after attempts is crucial, (3) that police and the
public should be educated about the suicidal and psychiatric
disorders and treatment, (4) organizations to which troubled
individuals may turn for information should be established, (5)
all suicide attempts should be reported to public health
officials and follow-up should be done, and (6) attention needs
to be paid to indirect life-threatening behavior patterns.
Bennett emphasizes that the most important suicide prevention
need, however, is public education regarding danger signs and
community mental health and other services.

3-005 Benson, Roger A., & Brodie, Donald C. (1975). Suicide by
overdoses of medicines among the aged. Journal of the American
Geriatrics Society, 23, 304-308.

The roles of physical illness and depression are discussed to establish the need to carefully prescribe (by the physician) and dispense (by the pharmacist) medications that the old may take to commit suicide. Method choice may often be made based on availability and the old frequently have barbiturates for insomnia. The authors suggest that a "safe supply" must be determined for each individual based on the evidence and circumstances. Clearly, useful drugs cannot be withheld simply because some elderly may take them to attempt suicide. The pharmacist is targeted, as the health professional most often contacted by the public, for attention to the potentially suicidal. In the summary the authors state that: "The problems of declining powers, physical and financial, and loss of status through retirement and death of loved ones require attitudes of adaptation more flexible than the older person can muster" (p. 307). They also suggest that other than treatment of mental and physical illness, that changing society's attitude toward the old "so that they may be accepted as a valuable, contributing segment of society, and not one that is segregated, pitied, and feared" (p. 308) may also aid in the prevention of suicide in the old.

3-006   Berdes, Celia. (1978). Social services for the aged dying and bereaved in international perspective (pp. 26-41, "Suicide and suicide prevention"). Washington, D.C.: International Federation on Ageing.

In addition to reviewing the literature on motivations to suicide in the old, a table of suicide data for 1971 are presented for 49 countries for those aged 65-74 and 75+ and comparing those aged 15-34 and 65+ for 6 countries. The author also notes two "modern types" of suicide which he calls (1) the "Van Dusen" and (2) "Tugend" types. The Van Dusens were a prominent elderly married couple who wanted to die together when one of them was faced with a painful or terminal illness and the other did not wish to live without the spouse. The other variety of modern suicide was named after Frank Tugend, the elderly retired coal miner who was slowly losing his control over his life and bodily functions as a result of an organic brain disorder. Rather than let death come as it may, he chose to take his teeth out and refuse food or drink. Three weeks later to the day he died. His grandsons, Mark and Dan Jury (1976, New York: Grossman) published a photographic essay of his life and especially the last months in the book Gramp. Berdes selects Sweden, Japan, and Israel for special consideration with regard to suicide among the old in those cultures. The review concludes with a lengthy presentation of prevention among the old. One of the problems of prevention is created by the isolation of the old which "makes it difficult to locate those in distress" (p. 32). Another is that telephone services for suicide prevention are typically not employed by the aged "because they fear dependence, are ignorant of the existence of such services, or are not accustomed to using the telephone" (p. 33). Two ideas to prevent elderly suicide are to use "senior citizens' centers as referral and screening centers" and "utilization of older people as volunteers in telephone crisis intervention centers" (p. 38) to ·increase the identification of the services as appropriate for and mindful of the problems of the old.

3-007 Breed, Warren, & Huffine, Carol L. (1979). Sex differences in suicide among older white Americans: A role and developmental approach. In Oscar J. Kaplan (Ed.), Psychopathology of aging (pp. 289-309). New York: Academic Press.

The authors focus on the tremendous sex difference in old age suicide among U.S. whites and attempt to integrate possible explanations by looking at existing theory and empirical data. They assume as a starting point that both life satisfaction and morale are inversely related to suicide and that factors which are related to high levels of satisfaction and morale will be associated with low levels of suicide. These authors integrate a great deal of research in gerontology and bring it to bear in understanding possible factors in elderly suicide and in the sex differences in particular. The model they suggest stresses the interaction between social and psychological factors and emphasizes as the primary factor adaptability. Adaptability is defined as the ability of the individual to survive crises physically, psychologically, and socially. The transition to old age is one of the crises of the life span. This chapter details differential socialization experiences of the sexes that make women more likely to be adaptable to changes than are men. Men are more likely to have difficulty in coping with the transition to old age, which includes the transition to the role of "retiree," and some will have the personality characteristics of rigidity and inflexibility. Those who are least flexible and adaptable are more likely to be high risks for suicide, especially under circumstances in which additional important elements are present such as physical illness, social isolation, economic difficulty, mental illness, etc.

3-008 Burnside, Irene M. (1981). Suicide in the aged person. In Irene M. Burnside (Ed.), Nursing and the aged (2nd ed.) (pp. 143-156). New York: McGraw-Hill. (1st ed., 1976, "Depression and suicide in the aged," pp. 165-181)

This chapter is written predominantly for a nursing audience, with a good mix of theory, statistics current at the time of the book's publication, research findings, practical and clinical information. The coverage includes forces that move the elderly toward life and suicide, direct and indirect self-destructive behavior, treatment and intervention. An assessment and management decision tree is also included as are 4 clinical vignettes that demonstrate various points made in the text. The chapter in the second edition of this book provides significantly expanded coverage of suicide from the first edition in which suicide was combined in a chapter with depression.

3-009   Busse, Ewald   W.,   &   Pfeiffer,   Eric.   (1969).   Functional
psychiatric disorders in old age.   In Ewald W. Busse & Eric
Pfeiffer (Eds.),   Behavior   and   adaptation   in   late   life
(pp. 183-235; especially pp. 221-224, "Suicide in old age").
Boston: Little, Brown.

This chapter briefly reviews the major findings on suicide among
the aged with respect to completed and attempted suicide, with
particular emphasis on the psychiatric diagnoses in completed
suicides and a discussion of prevention.   One statement that is
made regarding racial differences and trends is, however, given
current data (see McIntosh, 1985 and McIntosh & Santos, 1981,
reference 4-062)   incorrect: "Negroes have lower suicide rates
than white persons, but the pattern of increased suicide with
advancing   age is beginning to appear among Negro   men,
paralleling the pattern among white men" (p. 222).   While it is
accurate that blacks have lower rates than do whites, there has
been no tendency for black rates in old age to increase and
become more similar to those for whites with respect to changes
with age.   These authors also cite the lowest ratio of attempts
to completed suicide that can be found in the literature.   They
suggest that young people make 7 attempts for every completion
while the old attempt suicide in essentially the same numbers as
those who complete suicide.   With respect to prevention, the
authors suggest early and effective   treatment   of   mental
disorders, keeping old people active and involved socially, and
helping them through what is a temporary crisis so   that
adjustment can be made.

3-010   Cautela, Joseph R., & Mansfield, Linda. (1977).   A behavioral
approach   to geriatrics.   In   W. Doyle   Gentry   (Ed.),
Geropsychology: A model of training and clinical   service
(pp. 21-42, especially pp. 36-37, "An example of a behavioral
intervention: Prevention   of   suicide").   Cambridge,   MA:
Ballinger.

This article uses suicide as an example of how behavioral
intervention may be used with the elderly.   The authors state
that suicidal behavior may result from a combination of three
conditions: (1) aversive stimuli, (2)   lack   of   adequate
reinforcement, and (3) the learned response of escape.   If any
of these conditions are present, then suicide is seen as a
possibility. Suicide is viewed as the ultimate escape and may
be learned as a response from modeling or the lack of learning
adaptive responses to stress.   Suicide provides immediate escape
from the stress-producing situation that seems to have no other
way out.   The authors suggest several ways of eliminating a
learned escape response by removing aversive stimulation and
reinforcing incompatible responses.

3-011   Charatan, Fred B. (1979). The aged. In L. D. Hankoff & Bernice
Einsidler (Eds.), Suicide: Theory   and   clinical   aspects

(pp. 253–262). Littleton, MA: PSG Publishing.

The author considers the major factors in elderly suicide, including the sociological variables of sex, age, marital status, childlessness, religion, retirement and role loss, as well as physical health, alcohol and drug abuse, and psychiatric disorder. He begins the chapter with two examples that suggest fear of others in our current society as factors. Prevention efforts should be directed toward increasing the quality of life and value placed on the old. Political power and pressure are major forces in effecting such efforts. Treatment for suicidal thoughts is suggested to begin with hospitalization and the treatment of mental disorders followed after discharge by continuing psychiatric care and living in a sheltered environment such as a home for the elderly. In the case of attempts, the support of the family is encouraged.

3-012 Cutter, Fred. (1984).   Suicidal elders: Recognition and management. Clinical Gerontologist, 2(4), 66–68.

This brief article identifies the elderly most at risk to commit suicide: those who live alone, males, those with one or more previous attempts, people in terminal stages of a disease. The author suggests that differentiating between the high risk vs. the acute case is useful with respect to prevention. The author outlines the three circumstances in which the professional can legally intervene to prevent a suicide: (1) if the victim attempts to hurt him/herself in the practitioner's presence, (2) if the victim is young or immature, both mentally and emotionally, and (3) if the victim can be considered distraught so as to be incapable of rational choice.

3-013 Doyle, Polly. (1980). Grief counseling and sudden death: A manual and guide (pp. 129–151, Chapter 10, "Suicide--The young and the elderly," especially pp. 146–151, "Suicide and the elderly"). Springfield, IL: Thomas.

This brief coverage of elderly suicide includes the clues given by potentially suicidal aged individuals, depression, and stress. Community efforts to prevent elderly suicide should: (1) develop visitors programs using visitors who are trained to recognize suicidal elders, (2) utilize telephone services for crises, (3) provide suicide education and information about prevention, and (4) use senior centers for case finding.

3-014 Durkheim, Emile. (1951). Suicide: A study in sociology (translated by John A. Spaulding & George Simpson). New York: Free Press. (Originally published 1897 in French)

This work began the scientific study of suicide and presents theoretical notions that continue to generate contemporary research and discussion. While Durkheim did not focus exclusively on the elderly, but rather presented theoretical ideas he felt explained suicidal behavior more generally, there was consideration of the elderly. On page 29 the editor, George Simpson asks a series of questions regarding the elderly and their high suicide rates: Are deaths among the old more likely to be admitted as resulting from suicide? Does the high risk of degenerative disease in old age affect the elderly and their suicide likelihood? Is suicide self-murder when death is near anyway? Is the "social oblivion" the old encounter an invitation to return to "the kindly sleep of the unborn"?

Durkheim presents tabulations of data for many European countries during the 1800s by age. The increasing rates with increased age were apparent then as they are today, with highest rates in old age. Durkheim attempted to demonstrate that society is the decisive factor in suicide and is related to various social factors over which the individual has little control. He puts forth three types or explanations of why suicide occurs. Egoistic suicide results from the lack of integration into society by the individual. This is one of the major explanations for elderly suicide in Durkheim's theory. Altruistic suicide results from extreme integration of the individual into society. The individual here takes his/her own life for the good of the society. In some primitive societies the elderly would leave the group when they could no longer contribute, but this form of suicide does not seem to be a major pattern in contemporary society. Finally, anomic suicide was suggested to occur when there was a lack of regulation by the society upon the individual which resulted in a lack of clear norms for behavior. Such a state may exist among the newly retired elderly who are uncertain what their role now entails or following such events as divorce or widowhood. Durkheim points out that there can be mixtures of these social causes for suicide and the factors of egoism and anomie often occur together. Indeed, these two are the major forms in which elderly suicide seems to occur.

3-015   Foster, Betty G., & Burke, William J. (1985, November). Assessing and treating the suicidal elderly. Family Practice Recertification, 7(11), 33-45.

This article begins and ends with 5-item multiple choice tests of knowledge of elderly suicide. Following a brief presentation of the high risk demographic groups for suicide, social and psychological theoretical notions are considered. The remainder of the article discusses the recognition, treatment, and prevention of elderly suicide by physicians.

3-016   Friedeman, Joyce S. (1976, May/June). Cry for help: Suicide in the aged. Journal of Gerontological Social Work, 2(3), 28-32. (Revised version reprinted in Edna M. Stillwell (Ed.) (1980), Readings in gerontological nursing (pp. 131-136). Thorofare, NJ: Charles B. Slack.)

The article focuses on three areas: (1) The facts and fallacies of suicide in old age, e.g., the myth that the elderly are not capable of violent actions but are conservative and hesitant. (2) The effect of social structure on elderly suicide, and conversely the effect of their suicides on society. For example, losses in old age are highlighted, such as mobility, health, loved ones, mental acuity, and home. The author concludes that society en masse, is typically unaffected by elderly suicide due to the alienation and isolation of the elderly in "retirement" complexes. (3) The potential for intervention and prevention of elderly suicide by the nurse practitioner is outlined. The author states that "There is an unfortunate shortage of skilled professionals who have a specific interest in treating the dying, the self-destructive and suicidal, especially if the clients are aged" (p. 31).

3-017 Gage, Frances B. (1971). Suicide in the aged. American Journal of Nursing, 71, 2153-2155.

The author discusses the special needs of the elderly patient contemplating suicide and presents a case study. Techniques utilized to lessen suicide likelihood include encouraging the expression of anger and the exploration of discouragement while providing empathic support. The case study is clearly theoretically linked, culminating with a discussion of Erikson's integrity vs. despair stage (i.e., suicide as an unsuccessful emergence from the identity crisis of old age).

3-018 Gurland, Barry J., & Cross, Peter S. (1983). Suicide among the elderly. In Miriam K. Aronson, Ruth Bennett, & Barry J. Gurland (Eds.), The acting-out elderly (pp. 55-65). New York: Haworth Press.

This overview chapter presents information on high risk elderly, and the factors of mental illness, physical illness, and isolation in elderly suicide. The treatment of depression is discussed as well as less direct, suicidal equivalent behaviors. The efficacy of suicide prevention efforts is briefly noted. The authors note that suicide affects more than just the persons who kill themselves by stating that it also "blights those close to the victim" (p. 55). They "conjecture that, were care resources equal to those now devoted to cancer or the cardiovascular disorders to be directed at the social factors and individual vulnerabilities that precede suicide, the number of lives saved might rival that obtained in the more common cause of death" (pp. 55-56). They conclude their chapter by noting the importance of training mental health and other professionals regarding the elderly and suicide or depression, as well as the need to attack the problem of elderly suicide from social, economic, and medical fronts. Finally, they end their comments by stating that: "What can be projected for the future with respect to suicide rates in the elderly would seem to depend less on the changing demography than on what we and our policymakers do toward improving the quality of life and of health services for the elderly" (p. 65).

3-019 Kahne, Merton J., Olin, Harry S., Weisman, Avery D., Levin, Sidney, Berezin, Martin A., & Cath, Stanley H. (1973). Discussion [of suicide in the aging]. Journal of Geriatric Psychiatry, 6, 52-69.

Each of these individuals in turn present their thoughts regarding the case report of Haggerty (1973, reference 3-068) and the comments of Lettieri (1973, reference 4-051) about the prediction of suicidal risk in the aged. Many of the discussants indicate the limits of prediction from scale scores alone and the importance of clinical judgment in realizing the risk of suicide among individuals.

3-020 Kopell, Bert S. (1977, September). Treating the suicidal patient. Geriatrics, 32(9), 65-67.

Kopell suggests that suicide is a symptom of the stress of old age. Some of the factors he discusses with regard to suicide in the old are physical disability, poverty and economic status changes, and loneliness as well as psychological phenomena which are often adopted by the elderly to cope with aging. These phenomena, or defenses, are processes such as a concern with one's legacy, emotional disengagement from people and things, denial, rigidity, and projection. Kopell notes that while in younger persons these defenses may be seen as pathological, in the elderly they are adaptive coping mechanisms. He notes that the attempts by the old seem to be motivated by a desire to die rather than by the desire for sympathy and/or attention and that the suicidal old seem unlikely to seek mental health services. The importance of depression in elderly suicide is discussed along with methods of managing depression. The unique position of the physician to recognize the depressed and suicidal elderly and to refer them to community support services (e.g., mental health professionals) for areas outside the physician's competencies is discussed. As part of his conclusions, the author states that the motivation to suicide among some elderly may include the wish "to spare their families the economic devastation of providing medical care for their physical infirmities" or at other times it may be "a decision, based on reality, that life has little to offer" (p. 67).

3-021 Lesnoff-Caravaglia, Gari. (1983). Suicide in old age. In J. P. Soubrier & J. Vedrinne (Eds.), Depression and suicide: Aspects medicaux, psychologiques et socio-culturels (Proceedings of the 11th Congress of the International Association for Suicide Prevention, Paris, July 5-8, 1981) (pp. 581-586). New York: Pergamon Press.

This author discusses the "secret death of suicide" among the old. She notes that the environment is hostile to the old with negative societal attitudes and an emphasis on youth and health. The old encounter problems which they have never before encountered in life and with which they are most often ill prepared to deal. Fear of old age and the events which may

happen there may lead to suicide in old age. A "balance sheet"
approach to life may be taken to decide when the wish to die
outweighs the wish to live (see Portwood, 1978, reference
3-079). The old suffer many losses, possible dependence, loss
of mobility, illness and the fear of financial debts that will
leave surviving family members destitute. The author discusses
the clues to suicide that the old give. She states also that
with fewer contacts and the loss of significant others there are
fewer people to confide in and therefore, the clues of the old
are often not noticed.   "When the family or [institutional]
staff does not react to such clues, some of which may be quite
obvious, the older person's feeling that no one cares is
reinforced and promotes the decision to die" (p. 584).   Among
the concerns Lesnoff-Caravaglia raises is the danger of
suggested or encouraged suicide by the family of the elderly
person. The author also notes that there are few norms for the
individual who reaches old age and "They begin to strongly
suspect that the reason for the lack of norms is that society
really is not interested in them.   They begin to seriously
consider whether it matters that they live or die" (p. 584).

3-022 Leviton, Dan. (1973).   The significance of sexuality as a
       deterrent to suicide among the aged. Omega, 4, 163-174.

       Leviton hypothesizes that low sexuality (by definition, all that
       is associated with being a sexual person, the by-product of a
       loving relationship and the ability to enjoy oneself via coitus
       or other sexual behaviors) is highly correlated with suicidal
       desires, and that increased sexuality leads to decreases in
       suicidal ideation and behaviors. The following recommendations
       are made to improve/increase older persons' sexuality:
       recognition of personal attractiveness, recreational activity,
       encouragement of human relationships (nuturing, platonic,
       sexual), recognition of therapeutic aspects of healthy and
       functioning sexuality by hospital staff and administrators, and
       sexual functioning status evaluation incorporated into every
       medical workup.

3-023 Lyons, Michael J. (1984). Suicide in later life: Some putative
       causes with implications for prevention. Journal of Community
       Psychology, 12, 379-388.

       Lyons reviews factors related to suicide among the elderly and
       suggests preventive measures, especially primary prevention
       measures, to combat these factors.   He begins his review by
       suggesting that to be complete, any explanation of suicidal
       behavior must include both individual as well as environmental
       factors. Factors associated with aged suicide that are
       discussed include: physical illness, isolation and loss
       including the ramifications of retirement, depression and
       hopelessness, differential socialization practices for the
       sexes, economic conditions, attitudes and values both toward the
       elderly and on the part of the aged, and life satisfaction.
       Prevention measures to combat these factors include: the

provision of health care whether the old person can afford it or
not; education of medical personnel with respect to the effect
of illness on suicide risk; efforts to reduce isolation through
outreach programs, self-help groups for the bereaved, programs
that give the old a genuine opportunity for meaningful social
interaction, programs by widows that instruct widowers in
household skills, special efforts to insure that widowers are
active and not isolated;   the elimination of   mandatory
retirement, gradual retirement over a number of   years,
retirement planning and counseling, chances to use skills after
retirement, programs to teach new activities, college courses
offered to increase interests and teach skills; educational
programs about depression and its treatment;   programs that
provide financial security for the old, but not in the form of
services in place of income: and changes in male socialization,
in particular early in life.

3-024   McMordie, William R. (1984). The highest suicide risk--The
        elderly. In Elizabeth R. Prichard, Margot Tallmer, Austin
        H. Kutscher, Robert DeBellis, & Mahlon S. Hale (Eds.),
        Geriatrics and Thanatology (pp. 142-147). New York: Praeger.

        This very brief chapter overviews the levels, warning signs,
        treatment, and ethics of suicide. Its statistical presentation
        and many of the studies cited are quite dated and the
        information presented is primarily general rather than focused
        on the old. The need for postvention for professionals
        following a suicide completion is noted, but there is a glaring
        absence of any mention of the same need for the surviving family
        members.

3-025   Meerloo,   Joost   A. M. (1968).   Hidden   suicide.   In
        H. L. P. Resnik   (Ed.),   Suicidal behaviors: Diagnosis and
        management (pp. 82-89). Boston: Little, Brown.

        Hidden suicide (now more often called indirect self-destructive
        behavior   or subintentioned death) refers to the   various
        self-destructive paths through which individuals "steer toward
        death without being aware" (p. 82) of what they are doing.
        Several forms of hidden suicide are discussed, including drug
        addiction, accident-proneness, slow suicide through bodily
        dysfunction, and death that appears to be the result of
        another's death, which Meerloo refers to as   "contagious
        suicide." An interesting form of hidden suicide that Meerloo
        suggests but does not discuss in any detail is "suicide in the
        sexual fling at old age" (p. 88).

3-026   Miller, Marv. (1977). The physician and the older suicidal
        patient. Journal of Family Practice, 5, 1028-1029.

        This brief article attempts to draw the attention of physicians
        to their potential in suicide prevention among the old. It is
        pointed out that most suicidal people visit their physician
        shortly before their suicide or attempt and yet in many studies

the physicians apparently did not detect suicidal intent.
Miller contends that physicians may not detect the suicidal
because the topic of suicide is a taboo with which the
physician, like most other people, is uncomfortable and anxious.
Secondly, a lack of training in the recognition of danger signs
to suicide or intervention exists for the vast majority of
physicians. The physician also has the dilemma of drug
prescription when it is suspected that the older person may take
the drugs in an attempt to commit suicide. It is concluded that
physicians should go deeper than the physical complaints if they
are to see the suicidal intent that may be present in some of
their older patients.

3-027 Miller, Marv. (1979).   Suicide after sixty: The final
       alternative. New York: Springer. [The same adapted excerpt
       from this book appears in two articles entitled "Suicide after
       sixty" in Aging, November–December 1978, Nos. 289–290,
       pp. 28–31, and in Long Term Care and Health Administration
       Quarterly, 1979, 3, 92–97]

This book is a comprehensive review of the literature on
geriatric suicide. In the beginning chapters Miller presents
relevant facts and figures which dramatize the problem of
elderly suicide and overviews the literature on differences by
sex, race, religion, and other demographic variables.
Literature on elderly suicide is reviewed under the following
major headings: (1) familial and personal histories, (2) mental
and emotional problems, (3) physical illness and symptomatology,
(4) social factors, (5) precipitating factors and motives, (6)
means of lethality, (7) prevention, and (8) intervention.
Miller analyzes the multiple losses of aging and some of the
conditions which lead to alcoholism, depression, drug abuse,
mental illness, and suicide.

Miller provides 18 case examples from his previous research to
illustrate and highlight some of the different reactions to loss
(including the case in reference 3–071). He discusses the
important role of the physician in recognizing and preventing
suicide among the elderly.

In a comprehensive appendix Miller offers an excellent annotated
bibliography of sources for the reader (see also reference
2–003). He also includes a list of hard-to-find sources, some
of which are not in English.

3-028 Murray, Ruth B., Huelskoetter, M. Marilyn W., & O'Driscoll,
       Dorothy L. (1980). The nursing process in later maturity
       (pp. 549–575, Chapter 21, "Depression and suicidal tendencies in
       later maturity"). Englewood Cliffs, NJ: Prentice-Hall.

The literature on high risk individuals, motivations and clues
to elderly suicide are presented separately for suicide but most
of the chapter makes little differentiation between suicide and
depression. The majority of the chapter discusses primarily

depression in the old but special sections occur for suicide where appropriate. In a separate discussion on suicide prevention, the authors state that "Your supportive, warm relationship to the elderly senior is the greatest deterrent to suicide" (p. 570). Listening to the suicidal individual as well as providing support are encouraged as is the demonstration of caring for them as a person. The establishment of a promise from the person that they will contact you if they feel like killing themself is suggested.

3-029   Newquist, Deborah D. (1985). Voodoo death in the American aged: How beliefs about health and aging can affect the health of older people. In James E. Birren & Judy Livingston (Eds.), Cognition, stress and aging (pp. 111-133). Englewood Cliffs, NJ: Prentice-Hall.

Newquist discusses the sociocultural implications/definitions of age and how societies define the aging experience and thus the experience of aging. Attention is given to indirect, direct, and combined beliefs (in, for example, the power of hexes and spells) and their effects on health. Over time the cognitive processes in the belief-health relationship can produce two primary mechanisms: stress reaction and health-related behaviors. Voodoo death is conceptualized as death occurrences where culturally specific beliefs trigger emotional, behavioral, and social responses which, in turn, lead to negative health outcomes. In America, older persons are seen as dependent, needy, and dying (i.e., sick). Culturally, American aging is defined as a time of death and decline. To the extent that older persons subscribe to those beliefs, their health may be threatened, their longevity decreased. This conceptualization of voodoo death overlaps with the set of behaviors mentioned by others under the terms indirect self-destructive behavior and subintentioned death. Newquist suggests that our negative cultural views of aging and the old operate symbolically to negatively affect the health of these individuals as voodoo operates symbolically on its victims. To be old is to be sick and this decline metaphor becomes reality for the old. Newquist presents two models: the senescence model of health in which the older adult interprets physiological events as signs of aging, not illness and does not seek medical treatment; and the vanquished model in which older persons sees themselves as sick but just accept sickness as part of aging and seek no treatment.

3-030   Niccolini, Robert. (1973, May). Reading the signals for suicide risk. Geriatrics, 28, 71-72.

The author lists commonly used suicide-risk factors (i.e., age, sex, race, previous attempts, economic conditions, rural or urban environment, religious affiliation, and family history of suicide). Social isolation and depression are also addressed as meaningful factors. Physicians are advised to be aware of depressive symptomatology in their elderly clients.

3-031   Ofstein, Dennis, & Acuff,   F. Gene. (1979).   Durkheim   and
        disengagement: A causal model of aging suicide. Free Inquiry
        in Creative Sociology, 7, 108-117.

        This theoretical/conceptual article offers a causal model of
        aging suicide based on a synthesis of Durkheim's (reference
        3-014) egoistic model of suicide and a modification of the
        disengagement theory of aging. The model is theoretical and the
        specified paths are not differentiated by path coefficients. To
        support the proposed model the authors   review   existing
        literature and theory. They argue, for example, that factors
        which contribute to self-destructive behavior in the elderly
        include a weakening of social support and multiple losses.
        Retirement and widowhood are offered as examples of such losses.

        The model predicts the following relationship: forced
        disengagement leads to egoism which leads in turn to suicide,
        with an indirect link between forced disengagement and suicide.
        In support of their model the authors note that in societies in
        which the elderly are not readily disengaged, few suicide occur
        in late life. The authors call for empirical research to test
        the proposed theoretical model and to fill in path coefficients.

3-032   Osgood, Nancy J. (1982).   Suicide in the elderly: Are we
        heeding the warnings? Postgraduate Medicine, 72, 123-126, 128,
        130.

        Statistics on elderly American suicide are presented with
        special emphases on the overrepresentation of suicide and the
        highest suicide rates by age among the elderly.   Old age is
        described   as   a period of multiple losses accompanied by
        loneliness and severe depression. Distinctions are made between
        quality and quantity of life.   Several case examples   are
        presented to illustrate motivations and patterns of suicide
        among the elderly.   Warning signs, derived from the   case
        illustrations, are presented, including depression, increasing
        dependency, loss of social roles, diagnosis of terminal illness,
        major life changes, etc.   Depression, helplessness and
        dependency, loss of social roles and bereavement are discussed
        more thoroughly. Preventive measures for friends, relatives,
        physicians, ministers, and other caregivers are discussed.

3-033   Osgood, Nancy J. (1985a, March).   Identifying and counseling the
        suicidal geriatric patient.   Geriatric Medicine Today, 4(3),
        83-92.

        Many   suicides among the elderly can go   unreported   or
        unrecognized, yet the elderly possess the highest rate of
        suicide in America.   The elderly seem more serious about killing
        themselves than other age groups.   Often, physicians are the
        persons to whom the suicidal elderly turn (more than 75% of the
        elderly who commit suicide see a physician shortly before the
        act). Factors in elderly suicide include, among   others,
        depression, hopelessness, helplessness, bereavement and loss.

However, some elderly persons are more likely to commit suicide than others. White, urban, widowed or unmarried males are the most at risk for suicide in American society. Verbal, behavioral and syndromatic suicidal clues are discussed, as well as steps in assessing suicidal potential. Recommendations for counseling the geriatric patient include adapting treatment to the resources of the patient; taking a direct, active approach; being supportive and empathic; maintaining a problem-centered focus; maintaining coping mechanisms; and incorporating special catalysts (such as family photographs) into therapy.

3-034 Osgood, Nancy J. (1985b). <u>Suicide in the elderly: A practitioner's guide to diagnosis and mental health intervention</u>. Rockville, MD: Aspen Systems.

This book provides a comprehensive overview of the extent of the problem of elderly suicide and some of the causes, emphasizing the concepts of haplessness, hopelessness, and helplessness of the elderly. Theoretical and conceptual models and explanations for elderly suicide are also discussed in depth. Divided into three parts, Part Two focuses on detection and assessment of suicidal risk and lethality potential. Profiles of the "at risk" elderly are included. An overview of techniques and scales to assess depression, life satisfaction, loneliness, morale, and stress is provided, and actual scales are included in an appendix.

Drs. Mary Lou Melville and Dan G. Blazer contribute an excellent chapter on assessment of depression in the elderly. Suicide prevention and intervention are the focus in Part Three which includes chapters on reminiscence and life review therapy, the creative arts (drama, music, dance, and art), support groups, stress reduction and tension management. Drs. Soo Borson and Richard C. Veith contribute an expert chapter on pharmacological intervention. Two chapters, one in Part Two and one in Part Three, highlight the role of the caregiver in detection, prevention, and intervention. Each chapter contains an excellent list of references for the reader. The appendices include names and addresses of support groups for the widowed and those suffering from cancer, heart disease, or Alzheimer's Disease.

3-035 Osgood, Nancy J. (1985c). Suicides. In Erdman Palmore (Ed.), <u>Handbook of the aged in the United States</u> (pp. 371-390). Westport, CT: Greenwood Press.

In this overview chapter the author discusses major demographic factors in elderly suicide. Age, gender, race, marital status, social class and occupation, and living environment are addressed. A presentation is also made of major theoretical and conceptual models which have been offered to explain suicide. The cultural model focuses on differences between societies. The American emphasis on youth and beauty and negative stereotyping of the old are cited as factors accounting for the

high rate of suicide among the old in the U.S. Discussing the
sociological perspective, the author highlights Durkheim's
(reference 3-014) theory of social integration and suicide and
applies it to the case of elderly suicide. The psychological
perspective, which focuses on depression and despair as factors
in late life suicide, is examined. Finally, the stress model of
suicide is presented. Factors producing stress in older adults
are identified, and the literature relating stress to depression
and suicide is reviewed. In the conclusion, Osgood presents a
model of aging and suicide and a diagram of the suggested
relationships between the various factors.

3-036   Palmore, Erdman. (1975). The status and integration of the aged
in Japanese society. Journal of Gerontology, 30, 199-208.
(Reprinted in Jill S. Quadagno (Ed.) (1980), Aging, the
individual and society: Readings in social gerontology
(pp. 50-67). New York: St. Martin's Press.)

Japan is described as an exception to the rule of modernization
leading to declining social status of the elderly. Statistics,
observations, and interviews were collected in 1973. Standard
survey techniques of sample selection, interviewing procedures,
and data processing were used. Integration of Japanese elderly
is discussed in the three areas of family, workplace, and
community. Over 75% of Japanese aged 65 and over live with
their children (compared with 25% of America's senior citizens).
The economic necessity explanation of this phenomenon is
discounted. The elderly most often perform caretaker ("watcher
during absences") duties, particularly elderly women.
Additionally, Japanese elders serve as senior advisors on family
problems. Over half of the Japanese elderly men are active in
the work force (compared to less than one-third in America and
Britain). Two cultural traditions are described to account for
this (every able person should work as much and as long as
possible, and seniority and respect for the aged). Community
integration is evidenced by the membership in senior citizens'
clubs which are composed of over 50% of Japanese citizens over
65. These senior clubs provide community service, group
recreation, mutual support, study and action directed toward
helping elders, and are usually organized and subsidized by the
government. Visiting with neighbors and group sight-seeing
trips are also popular with the Japanese elderly.

Respect for elders is evidenced by their continued ties with the
family, the workplace, and the community, as well as in the
honorific language used in speaking to or about elders.
Governmental programs for the elderly include health
examinations, homes for the aged, family foster care, free
medical services, home helpers, etc. Vertical societal
structure and filial piety are presented as the roots of respect
for Japanese elders. Relatively small and slow declines in the
status of Japanese elderly are acknowledged, although the author
predicts some continued decline in elderly status with
increasing modernization. The relatively high suicide rate

among Japanese aged is also addressed. While some would say
that high suicide rates are indicative of lower social
integration, the author again points to a cultural explanation:
suicide rates are higher in Japan at all ages and is seen as an
honorable solution to personal difficulties.

3-037   Patterson, Robert D., Abrahams, Ruby, & Baker, Frank. (1974,
        November). Preventing self-destructive behavior. Geriatrics,
        29(11), 115-121.

The authors discuss varied self-destructive behaviors in the
elderly and provide recommendations for intervention. Suicide
rates in the elderly can be reduced through physicians' accurate
diagnoses and treatment of depression. Relational losses,
despair, and hypochondriacal concerns are discussed in relation
to depression. Subintentional self-destructive behaviors are
presented, including weight abnormalities, neglect of routine
medical examinations, heavy smoking, not adhering to medical
treatment, not planning for medical emergencies, and alcoholism.
Although physical survival is important, the ultimate goal is
physical survival coupled with meaningful psychological life.
Means of reducing/avoiding unnecessary psychological stress
through thoughtful planning are discussed.

3-038   Pavkov, Janet. (1982). Suicide and the elderly. Ohio's Health,
        34(1), 21-28.

In this article the author focuses on recognition and prevention
of suicide in the elderly. A discussion of ten major myths and
ten major facts about suicide in the old is presented. The
factors of depression, haplessness, helplessness, and
hopelessness, as well as the loss/stress model of elderly
suicide are considered. A mental health profile and depression
checklist which can be used in assessment by practitioners is
included. Several therapeutic treatment goals regarding highly
lethal older adults are listed.

3-039   Payne, Edmund C. (1975). Depression and suicide. In John
        G. Howells (Ed.), Modern perspectives in the psychiatry of old
        age (pp. 290-312). New York: Brunner/Mazel.

Suicide as a public health and clinical problem is
underestimated by the general public and the medical profession,
particularly with regard to the aging population. Life
circumstances and intrapersonal factors leading to suicide in
the elderly are reviewed in an attempt to better understand
elderly suicide and to explore optimal management and treatment
of the suicidal individual. Investigations of suicidal
phenomena have been characterized by two theoretical stances:
the sociological point of view and the clinical point of view.
The sociological viewpoint has traditionally purported that
suicide is explainable in terms of the individual's relationship
to his/her social group, while the clinical approach is based on
the study of individual cases. The clinical approach frequently

focuses on mental illness to the exclusion of psychosocial environmental factors in evidence from the sociological approach. As suicide is a complex act composed of multiple factors, the optimal explanatory model would integrate clinical and sociological viewpoints.

The sociological approach to suicide was pioneered by Emile Durkheim (reference 3-014) in the late 1800s and early 1900s. Durkheim's work established that suicide is not a disease, and not solely the outcome of mental illness, even though a close relationship exists between suicide and depression. Social and psychological factors merge in a complex fashion to find their expression in suicide. These factors are thought to vary with age. Those factors correlated with suicide and aging are discussed in detail and include: statistics (including sex differences) on elderly suicide, occupational and economic factors, loss and loneliness, and societal attitudes toward the elderly.

The clinical approach to suicide has focused on the link between depressive illness and suicide. Affective disorders have become an exciting research area, although the validity of the dichotomous classification of depression (endogenous vs. reactive) has been seriously questioned. The relationship of physical illness to suicide in the elderly is less clear. The decision to end one's life rather than await the termination of a fatal illness may be a rare event. More frequently, the illness is experienced as debilitatingly stressful, and leads to loss of activity, increased dependency, and social isolation. Psychotherapy accounts of work with suicidal persons are rare. Consequently, generalizations about emotional stability and subjective experiences of these patients are suspect.

Physicians' role in the recognition of suicidal behavior is discussed and attention given to the fact that many suicidal elders visit a physician before committing the act. Physicians are urged to be aware of their own emotional reluctance to respond to (and recognize) distressing emotions in patients; to be aware of suicidal signs; to evaluate the suicidal risk, and if necessary, refer to mental health professionals; and to involve the family to strengthen emotional supports. The advantages and disadvantages of hospitalization or outpatient management are discussed. Treatment methods are discussed and include: keeping the patient alive until treatment can be effective, and social intervention (amelioration of the psychological issues contributing to the patient's depression).

3-040   Pelizza, John J. (1979). Suicide in the elderly: Can it be prevented? Long Term Care and Health Services Administration Quarterly, 3(2), 85-91.

The author discusses demographic factors in suicide (i.e., age, sex, race, economic status, marital status, physical health). Durkheim's (reference 3-014) basic categories of suicide (egoistic, altruistic, anomic) are described and a newer term, "social disorganization," is presented as a more current equivalent for anomic suicide. Retirement, loss of family interaction, and the resulting depression are discussed as examples of the disorganizing effects of later life. Suicide indicators (depression, withdrawal, isolation, etc.) are listed and several recommendations made for prevention of depression. These recommendations include: family involvement, pre-retirement programs, and utilization of social service agencies including public health services. The critical variable in staving off depression and suicidal ideation, according to this author, is increasing social interaction opportunities.

3-041   Pfeiffer, Eric, & Busse, Ewald W. (1973). Mental disorders in later life--Affective disorders, paranoid, neurotic, and situational reactions. In Eric Pfeiffer & Ewald W. Busse (Eds.), Mental illness in later life (pp. 107-144). Washington, D.C.: American Psychological Association.

Particularly on pages 123-126, the authors discuss several factors in elderly suicide (i.e., race, sex, marital status, psychiatric diagnosis). Recommendations for suicide prevention revolve around early and effective treatment of psychiatric disorders. Paranoid disorders are especially discussed due to the high incidence of paranoid reactions among the aged.

3-042   Pollinger-Haas, Ann, & Hendin, Herbert. (1983). Suicide among older people: Projections for the future. Suicide and Life-Threatening Behavior, 13, 147-154.

Given the trend for the positive relationship between the size of a cohort group and suicide rates, and the fact that the distress level of a cohort group tends to remain fairly constant over the lifetime, the authors attempt to make some predictions regarding possible suicide trends among future generations of older people. By using demographic projections of age groups up to the year 2040, they propose that suicide rates among the elderly will continue to increase as the elderly population becomes a larger proportion of the total population and high risk cohorts become older.

3-043   Poulos, J. (1971, July). The geriatric suicide. Bedside Nurse, 4, 24-26.

The link between depression and old age, and historical theories discussing old age melancholy are presented, as well as the relationship between depression and suicide and the severity of intent among elderly suicide attempters. Warning signs of suicide (loss of loved one, previous suicidal behavior, psychiatric disorders, etc.) are described. The nurses' role in encouraging continued social involvement, and making personal contact with the elderly patient is given. The need for reinforcement of self-worth and awareness of social psychological problems is emphasized.

3-044 Rachlis, David. (1970, Fall).   Suicide and loss adjustment in
the aging. Bulletin of Suicidology, No. 7, pp. 23-26.

Rachlis notes that few services to specifically prevent elderly
suicide have been established and the old do not often utilize
the existing services, particularly telephone crisis services.
The self-reliance of the old, especially among males, result in
reluctance to use such services because they feel they should
solve their own problems.   The author describes old age as
"mostly a growing-down process" (p. 23) to indicate the large
number of losses that occur.   The accumulation of losses alone
are not sufficient for suicide, however, and the importance of
the personal response is noted. Rachlis suggests some "creative
approaches" to reach and prevent suicide among the old: (1)
Senior citizen centers could be used to identify the suicidal
old, refer for help, and provide support.   In essence then, the
senior centers could become the suicide prevention centers for
the old with properly trained professionals and members.   (2)
"Research is needed to explore the linkage between 'retirement
shock' and suicide" (p. 24).   (3) A predictive instrument needs
to be developed so that the suicidal may be identified and
intervention may be made appropriately. Rachlis suggests that
this instrument also be constructed such that laypersons could
use it.   One element of this instrument might be the
identification of the losses mentioned in this article.   The
author suggests several reasons why we should make genuine
efforts to prevent elderly suicide.   Humanitarian reasons as
well as the repayment of the debt society owes the old are two
such reasons, but Rachlis suggests also that the old have
economic potential that has been neglected and ignored.   Their
experience makes them particularly prepared to do many jobs
where there is a shortage of personnel (child care, teaching
skills, home maintenance, etc.).   Additionally, "helping the
aging now is in a sense buying insurance for the younger
generations. Supportive health and social welfare services
developed today will provide security in the later years for the
presently young and middle-aged. They will enter later life
with assurance that help will be available to deal with the
inevitable losses of aging" (p. 25). He suggests that efforts
equal to those currently made to educate youth be made to
preventing self-destruction among the old "who built the
comforts we now enjoy" (p. 26).

3-045 Resnik, H. L. P., & Cantor, Joel M. (1970).   Suicide and aging.
Journal of the American Geriatrics Society, 18, 152-158.
(Reprinted in V. M. Brantl & M. R. Brown (Eds.) (1973), Readings
in gerontology (pp. 111-117). St. Louis: Mosby. Reprinted in
Steven Steury & Marie L. Blank (Eds.) (1977), Readings in
psychotherapy with older people (pp. 215-219).   Washington,
D.C.: USGPO, DHEW Publication No. (ADM) 78-409.)

The authors discuss the suicide rates of whites in contrast to the nonwhite population and the decrease since 1950 in the number of elderly suicides. A presentation is made of the theoretical considerations of Freud, Menninger, Jung, and Durkheim, followed by a discussion of suicide potential indicators (prior suicidal behavior, bereavement and loss, psychiatric disorders, serious physical illness, putting possessions in order, and suicidal threats). Intervention strategies of taking action and involving others are outlined and discussed. It is apparently in this article that the often repeated statement that "the aged comprise 9 per cent [at that time] of the population, yet they contribute 25 per cent of the suicides" (p. 153) began.

3-046   Richman, Joseph. (1984). Psychotherapy and family therapy with the suicidal elderly [Abstract]. In Cynthia R. Pfeffer & Joseph Richman (Eds.), Proceedings of the 15th annual meeting of the American Association of Suicidology (pp. 84–86). Meeting held in New York City, April 1982. Denver: American Association of Suicidology.

The author states three contentions in this brief summary paper: (1) The vast majority of suicides are preventable, even in advanced old age. (2) The suicidal elderly can be helped to live a meaningful and satisfying existence. And (3) Psychotherapy, especially family therapy, can contribute in a major way to this outcome.

The author argues that the relatives of a suicidal older adult are the best treatment resources and can help prevent the suicide. He further identifies three factors which increase the risk of suicide in the old: ego weakening states, isolation, and interpersonal factors. Richman refers to a 1975 study he conducted in which he found that family dissension was a major factor in the great majority of suicide attempts of the young and the old.

A brief discussion is made of the goals and methods of evaluation and treatment of suicidal elders. The goals are to increase mutual regard and the family can be made a self-help group. Methods of evaluation and treatment include an individual interview and assessment of the suicidal person and each relative, a diagnostic family interview, rating of suicidal risk, intervention such as family therapy, and contacting and working with doctors, social workers and other professionals.

3-047   Sainsbury, Peter. (1961). Suicide in old age. Proceedings of the Royal Society of Medicine, 54, 266–268.

In this brief paper Sainsbury reviews the literature on various social and psychiatric factors related to suicide of the old and discusses prevention. Summarizing existing statistics on suicide and age, he notes that suicide rates increase sharply with age, the rise in suicide rates in late life holds true for nearly all nations except pre-war China, the suicide rates for males has been declining in the past 50 years, and female rates, especially for the old, have been increasing.

Reviewing the literature on psychiatric factors, Sainsbury discusses the role of depression, illness, loneliness, and bereavement. Pathological depression precedes suicide in about half of the cases. Bereavement more often precedes suicide in late life. Sainsbury also discusses crises in personal relationships as a factor in late life suicide.

To prevent suicide among the old, Sainsbury recommends that all suicidal intent be taken seriously, that apparently minor ailments be corrected, that attitudes toward life, death, and suicide be discussed openly and frankly, and taking necessary social measures to make older people feel they are useful and have a real place in the community.

3-048   Santos, John F., Hubbard, Richard W., & McIntosh, John L. (1983). Mental health and the minority elderly. In Lawrence D. Breslau & Marie R. Haug (Eds.), Depression and aging: Causes, care, and consequences (pp. 51-70). New York: Springer.

This chapter reviews the literature relating to mental health and depression among ethnic/minority elderly and ethnic differences in cognitive and personality characteristics that might influence reactions to a therapist, therapy, and the use of mental health services. The authors begin by noting the lack of relevant literature on minorities and the many myths which prevail.

The literature on depression in the black elderly is contradictory; however, marital problems, deaths in the family, and other environmental situations which may stimulate depression have been found to be more frequent for blacks than whites. There is general agreement in the literature that elderly blacks are low suicide risks, especially when compared to young blacks or elderly whites.

Studies of depression among Hispanic elderly reveal higher levels of depression for Hispanics than for whites or blacks. Although results are contradictory, most studies have shown suicide to be more prevalent among young than old Hispanics. The need for bilingual/bicultural therapists is noted.

The depression literature for Asian-American elders is nonexistent. The authors describe the plight of these individuals as worse than that of the black or Hispanic elderly. The Asian elderly are few in number and have more cultural, language, educational, and economic barriers. They have been found to have the least contact with social service and government agencies of any group. The suicide rate for Asian-American elderly is lower than that for whites following great declines from the 1940s and 1950s.

As for most other minorities, little literature on depression and personality characteristics exists for Native American elderly. Tribal group differences are large and it may be inappropriate to generalize based on studies of one or some tribes. Alcohol tends to be a major factor in suicide among this group. Native American elderly have much lower rates of suicide than young Native Americans and the white elderly.

The differences between ethnic/minority groups are discussed. Despite differences, however, all groups share in common a reluctance to enter therapy, reluctance to disclose in therapy, and high drop out rates. The authors call for more research into the problem. [Further detailed discussion of suicide counseling and intervention with minorities may be found in McIntosh & Santos, 1984, Chapter 7 in Corrine L. Hatton & Sharon M. Valente (Eds.), Suicide: Assessment and Intervention (2nd ed.) (pp. 175-194). Norwalk, CT: Appleton-Century-Crofts.]

3-049   Seiden, Richard H. (1981). Mellowing with age: Factors influencing the nonwhite suicide rate. International Journal of Aging and Human Development, 13, 265-284.

Seiden explores the demographics of suicide as a means of comparing white and nonwhite suicide. Although there are exceptions within the specific groups which comprise the nonwhite population, suicide rates for nonwhites peak in young adulthood and decline to low levels in old age whereas among whites rates increase with age to highest levels in old age. Seiden proposes six hypotheses for possible explanation of the differences in suicide rates by age for white and nonwhite populations. Three hypotheses are statistical in nature (differential life expectancy, selective screening, deviant burnout), and three are sociocultural (role and status, traditional values, age-specific motives for suicide). He concludes that nonwhite elderly persons may experience old age as a reward in itself, find life worth living and are more likely to show higher levels of morale than whites, as evidenced by their lower suicide rates. The level of institutionalized racism in America prevents nonwhites from gaining occupational power and authority; therefore, the loss of status resulting from retirement may not be the same for nonwhite populations as for the white population. Finally, Seiden points to the family structure of nonwhite populations which "by necessity as much as design" provides a sense of belonging and status for the elderly nonwhite.

3-050   Seiden, Richard H. (1983, November). Suicide among the young and elderly. Paper presented at the annual meeting of the Gerontological Society of America, San Francisco.

In this presentation, made as part of a symposium on elderly suicide, Seiden lists proposed areas of shared conflict between the young and the elderly in an attempt to increase understanding of the relatively higher suicide rates in these two groups. Physiological changes, identity conflicts, problems with employment/underemployment, economic hardship, powerlessness, sexuality, and drug use are described as shared conflict areas. The differences between objective and subjective success are discussed, as well as the differences between black/nonwhite and white suicide.

3-051   Sendbuehler, J. M. (1977). Suicide and attempted suicide among the aged [Editorial]. Canadian Medical Association Journal, 117, 418–419. [Correspondence: W. W. Blue, 1977, 117, 418–419. C. H. Cahn, 1977, 117, 1136.]

The author subscribes to a comprehensive method of study described as "a building-up of statistics." The intent is to provide information broad enough about suicides to encompass epidemiological, psychiatric, and psychological bases. Although suicide attempters have many of the same demographic descriptors as the normal population (i.e., race, age, sex, marital status, ethnic group, religion, social class), there are variables which are not so often included in discussion of suicidal tendencies. Physical illness, psychopathological disorders, and multiple losses are often part of the older suicidal individual's history as well. Organic brain syndrome, although mentioned infrequently as a precursor of suicide, tends to interfere with successful completion of the suicidal act due to clouding of the sensorium. Generally, individuals with psychotic symptoms fail in their suicide attempts. The author raises the question of whether this leads to "survival of the unfittest" and concludes unsuccessful suicides, hampered by organic brain syndrome or psychotic thought processes, should be viewed as a distorted call for help.

3-052   Shamoian, Charles A. (1984). Suicide in the elderly: A clinical overview [Abstract]. In Cynthia R. Pfeffer & Joseph Richman (Eds.), Proceedings of the 15th annual meeting of the American Association of Suicidology (pp. 67–69). Meeting was held in New York City, April 1983. Denver: American Association of Suicidology.

In this short synopsis the author presents some major facts and figures on elderly suicide. He notes that 20–25% of the old have severe psychopathology requiring intervention, however, the vast majority never receive any treatment. According to Shamoian, anxiety reactions, affective disorders, alcoholism and drug abuse are some of the more common functional disorders experienced by older adults. Death of a spouse, physical illness, alcohol or drug abuse, depression, and past history of suicide attempts are major factors in elderly suicides. The author suggests that medical and psychiatric exams are an absolute minimum in evaluating any elderly individual. The article also contains a brief description of psychopharmacologicals such as antidepressants and antianxiety agents and their use with the elderly.

3-053 Shneidman, Edwin S. (1965, May). Preventing suicide. American
Journal of Nursing, 65(5), 111-116. (Reprinted in Jack P. Gibbs
(Ed.) (1968), Suicide (pp. 255-266). New York: Harper & Row.
Reprinted in Bulletin of Suicidology, December 1980, No. 4,
pp. 19-25. Reprinted in Edwin S. Shneidman, Norman L. Farberow,
& Robert E. Litman (Eds.) (1970), The psychology of suicide
(pp. 429-440). Reprinted in Brent Q. Hafen & Eugene J. Faux
(Eds.) (1971), Self-destructive behavior: A national crisis
(pp. 256-265). Minneapolis, MN: Burgess. Reprinted in Robert
F. Weir (Ed.) (1977), Ethical issues in death and dying
(pp. 363-373). New York: Columbia University Press. Reprinted
as The warning signs of suicide," in Marv Miller (Ed.) (1982),
Suicide intervention by nurses (pp. 31-45). New York:
Springer.)

The major issue in suicide prevention is diagnosis and
identification. The author presents several assumptions:
suicide attempters wish to be rescued; suicide prevention
depends on the active and forthright behavior of the potential
rescuer; individuals about to attempt suicide are very
conscious of their intentions; most suicides stem from
isolation or intolerable emotions; suicide results from an
internal complex debate; and in almost every suicide there are
prodromal clues. Although these warning signs were written
originally for nurses, the information is easily generalized.
The basic prodromal clues seem to be common to all age groups
and are suggested by Shneidman to be of four broad types:
verbal, behavioral, situational, and syndromatic. Verbal clues
may be direct ("I'm going to kill myself.") or indirect
("Goodbye, I won't be here when you get back."). Behavioral
clues as well may be direct (a past suicide attempt) or indirect
(e.g., putting affairs in order). Situational clues revolve
around stressful situations in the person's life, such as
mutilative surgery, unemployment, loss, etc. Finally, the
syndromatic clues are circumstances in which a cluster of
symptoms, when put together, comprise a syndrome. Syndromatic
clues suggested in the article are depression, defiance,
disorientation, and dependent-dissatisfied. Suicide impacts
patients, staff, coworkers, family and friends. Even unclear
suspicions of suicide potential in another person should be
addressed. Professionals are encouraged to be aware of their
own reactions to certain patients (i.e., are you willing to
"hear" this patient's cries for help?).

3-054 Shneidman, Edwin S. (1971). Suicide in the aged. In Richard
Davis (Ed.), The doctor and the dying patient (pp. 1-6). Los
Angeles: University of Southern California. (Reprinted in
Richard H. Davis (Ed.) (1973), Dealing with death (pp. 25-32).
Los Angeles: University of Southern California.)

Suicide is conceptualized as "tenaciously dyadic" in that the
suicidal person always brings in the "significant other"
(whether the significant other is a life-saver or suicidogenic
is a question the therapist must answer). The pervasive

ambivalence of suicide is discussed and it is suggested that
while the suicide has rights, the surviving family members have
rights also. Shneidman also defines and discusses the concepts
of premature death, pacific death, appropriate death,
intentioned death, subintentioned death, and non-intentioned
death. It is suggested that death certificates should take into
account these three potential roles one can take in their own
death--intentioned, subintentioned, non-intentioned. The three
levels of "vention" in suicide (prevention, intervention, and
postvention) are also considered as is the concept of
psychological autopsy which may be undertaken to determine the
mode of death but may also be actively therapeutic for the
survivors. In the final section an argument is made that
suicide may be an "appropriate" death that is best for both the
victim and survivors. It is also noted that many deaths of
older persons are subintentioned. Such deaths take the form of
refusal to eat, not following important medical regimens, having
fatal "accidents," etc.

3-055   Shulman, Kenneth. (1978). Suicide and parasuicide in old age:
A review. Age and Ageing, 7, 201-209.

The author points out that compared to other age groups, among
the elderly parasuicides (suicide attempters) and completed
suicides more closely resemble each other. Therefore, attempts
in this group should be taken seriously no matter how
gesture-like or manipulative they appear. The high rate of
suicide in the old is noted as is the lack of attention to the
elderly in the psychiatric literature. The author identifies
the major factors in geriatric suicide to be depression,
hypochondriasis, bereavement, social isolation, and physical
illness. An excellent review of the literature on each factor
is provided. The article concludes with a schematic model of
suicide and parasuicide in late life which shows the
relationship between factors.

3-056   Stenback, Asser. (1980). Depression and suicidal behavior in
old age. In James E. Birren & R. Bruce Sloane (Eds.), Handbook
of mental health and aging (pp. 616-652). Englewood Cliffs, NJ:
Prentice-Hall. (Reprinted under the title "Suicidal behavior in
old age" in K. Warner Schaie & James Geiwitz (Eds.) (1982),
Readings in adult development and aging (pp. 369-384). Boston:
Little, Brown.)

This chapter provides an overview of depression and suicide in
late life. Depression is defined and primary and secondary
symptoms are discussed. The etiology of depression is the focus
of a second part of the chapter. In this section psychological,
biological, social, and cultural factors are outlined. The
multiple losses (personal, biological, emotional, social,
financial) of old age are a central theme in the etiology of
depression. Sections on varieties of depressive disorders and
other affective disorders are followed by a section presenting a
schematic model of depression. This model and each of its

components (environment, the individual, significant life events, biological and psychological reactions) are discussed in detail and pertinent literature is reviewed.

The course and prognosis of depressive illness in late life are analyzed in another section of the chapter. Factors which are associated with a favorable prognosis are: age under 70, positive family history, extraverted personality, social ties and activities extending beyond the family. Unfavorable factors were physical senility or physical defects and disabilities. In old age depression increasingly manifests itself in somatic symptoms. Closely related to this increased somatization is the depletion state, a state of emptiness, decline, helplessness, and loss of interests and energy. Therapy for depression is considered next. Crisis intervention and brief therapy are among those described.

The final section of the chapter dealt with suicide and attempted suicide. Factors identified as contributing to suicide and suicide attempts included: mental illness, physical illness, social isolation and loneliness, marital status (being unmarried), retirement, living alone or moving, poverty, and social disorganization. The literature for each factor was briefly reviewed. The author concludes that factors promoting suicide among the elderly may be grouped into five causes: general and age-specific losses; an egoistic or excessively individualistic personality; a society unable to integrate older members; a personality trait of resolving problems through action; and a suicide-promoting environment, either personal or cultural. Treatment to decrease suicide was suggested and drug treatment, psychotherapy, and sociotherapy were recommended. Macrosocial measures such as improved housing and higher income for the old were also suggested.

3-057   Stengel, E. (1965). The prevention of suicide in old age. Zeitschrift fur Praventivmedizin, 10, 474-481.

The author addresses the issue of elderly suicide and discusses special circumstances of the aged which may contribute to increased suicidal behavior (i.e., illness, social conditions including economic factors). Social isolation is presented as the most important etiological factor in aged suicide. Recommendations for prevention include improvement of medical services and inclusion in the work force.

3-058   Strahan, Charles, Jr. (1980). The retired person: Boredom, fears and suicide. Delaware Medical Journal, 52, 497-501.

The focus of this article is on the retired person who cannot cope with retirement. For some retired individuals life becomes days of emptiness and worry with too much time on their hands. The case of Mr. Y, who became bored and depressed after he retired from his job at a chemical firm, is presented. His case demonstrated some of the problems retirees face: boredom, fears, loss and mourning, and suicide. The author suggests that early recognition of the shocking effect of retirement and proper intervention techniques can prevent suicide among older retired individuals.

3-059 Tideiksaar, Rein. (1978). On suicide and the aging [Letter]. American Journal of Public Health, 68, 782–783.

This brief commentary reviews the work of others on elderly suicide and discusses the problem of concealed suicide and underreporting. The author suggests that we look more closely at accidental deaths as concealed suicides. In the final section the author suggests that suicide rates are an indicator of poor mental health among our elderly and calls for the development of greater accuracy in suicide statistics and proper therapeutic intervention.

3-060 Tideiksaar, R. (1979). Suicide in the elderly [Letter]. American Family Physician, 19(3), 28–30.

The author cites statistics on the high rate of suicide among the old and points out that suicide is not a cry for help in this age group. He claims that retirement is a factor in elderly suicide as are physical decline and illness. It is noted that the elderly who kill themselves generally consult a doctor shortly before their lethal act, and it is recommended that family physicians be especially alert to the possibility of suicidal ideation among their elderly patients.

3-061 Tomorug, E. (1970). Biological crises and suicide. In Richard Fox (Ed.), Proceedings: Fifth international conference for suicide prevention, London, September 24–27, 1969 (pp. 194–195). Vienna: International Association for Suicide Prevention.

The author begins by noting the alarming increase in suicidal attempts by women and juveniles. Depression is at the root of suicidal behavior, according to the author, and most depression is the result of some biological crisis. Puberty is cited as a period of such crisis in adolescence, and premenstrual tension and menstruation were important in suicide attempts of young girls. Old age is a time of biological crises, with an excessive suicidal tendency. Retirement adds to the risk of suicide among elderly males. Finally, the burden of prevention rests on psychiatry, and the author calls for the establishment of more suicide prevention centers.

3-062 Trout, Deborah L. (1980). The role of social isolation in suicide. Suicide and Life-Threatening Behavior, 10, 10–23.

Social isolation is defined as a state in which interpersonal contacts and relationships are disrupted or nonexistent. The author reviews the literature on the role of social isolation in suicide. Theoretical views on suicide and social isolation are discussed briefly, and the concept of methods of measuring social "integration" and "isolation" is introduced. Subjective and objective measures of an individual's social isolation are concluded to be necessary in the study of the relationship between social isolation and suicide. Sainsbury's (1955, Suicide in London, London: Chapman & Hall) contention that "people who lead isolated lives, deprived of contact either with family, friends, or religious community, are most exposed to the risk of suicide" has been supported by varied investigators. The author concludes that social uninvolvement, particularly solitary living, appears to be related to suicidal behavior. Research results indicating suicidal individuals typically have had problems with social relationships and loneliness since childhood, including communication problems, progressive alienation, gradual withdrawal from social contacts, and a sense of isolation from the rest of society are cited. Social isolation is depicted as a primary and direct factor in suicide. Among recommendations made for intervention are: the dissolution of the individual's pain through the establishment of an accepting and sustaining human contact; increased involvement in social activities; and the need for supportive and educational public programs to deal with social isolation as a societal problem. The problem of social isolation becomes a particularly important issue with respect to elderly suicide because the old are the most likely population to be living alone and in socially isolated circumstances.

3-063 Veevers, J. E. (1973). Parenthood and suicide: An examination of a neglected variable. Social Science and Medicine, 7, 135-144.

Marital status, sex, age, and race have been demonstrated to be systematically related to suicide rates. However, little research has focused on the variable of parenthood as a protector against suicide. The author explores the relationship between childlessness and suicide in an attempt to determine the relationship between parenthood and suicide rates. Several assumptions are made: Parents are assumed to have higher degrees of social integration than non-parents due to possessing both marital and parental social bonds; the psychological characteristics that lead to the decision to avoid parenthood may also lead to suicidal impulses (nonparents are generally considered neurotic, maladjusted and emotionally disturbed); and without the benefits of parenthood, it is difficult, if not impossible, to achieve full social and psychological maturity that would lessen the likelihood of suicide. Durkheim's and Halbwach's research on parental status and suicide (i.e., no children) are presented. Statistics indicating suicide rates are higher among single than married persons are noted. The author hypothesizes that persons with sound mental health are both less likely to commit suicide and most likely to get and stay married. On the other hand, married persons (through the benefits of marriage) are more likely to be integrated into more social groups. Divorced versus widowed persons rates of suicide are also compared, with rates among the divorced higher. The

author hypothesizes that divorced persons are perceived as
failures and the psychological stresses associated with these
failures are associated with higher suicide rates.
Additionally, the divorce process, in and of itself, may be
selective of persons whose psychological stability and
adjustment are less satisfactory than those persons not choosing
divorce as an option. With child custody laws favoring the
mother, fathers deprived of their children would be more likely
to commit suicide.

Widowed persons, in contrast to the divorced, are not perceived
as to blame for the lack of a spouse. The hypothesis is made
that widowed persons' suicide rates would be low until all
children leave home and the "empty nest syndrome" develops. The
author concludes by suggesting that variations in suicide rates
traditionally attributed to varying marital status may be more
accurately attributed to different parental statuses. With
respect to the elderly, Veevers leaves unresolved the issue of
adult children and their roles in the lives of their elderly
parents and the effect that might have on the suicidal potential
of the aged parent. This issue remains to be resolved through
further research.

3-064   Waldron, Ingrid. (1976). Why do women live longer than men?
        Social Science and Medicine, 10, 349-362.

Mortality rates for men are 60% higher than for women in
contemporary society. Of this sex difference in mortality, 40%
is attributed to arteriosclerotic disease which occurs twice as
often in men as women. More cigarette smoking and Type A
behavior (i.e., competitive and aggressive) are thought to be
two reasons for the larger incidence of arteriosclerotic disease
in men. Of the remaining sex diffential in mortiality, 33% is
due to men's higher rates of suicide, fatal motor vehicle and
other accidents, respiratory cancer, emphysema and cirrhosis of
the liver. Males in our society are expected and encouraged to
be "tough, strong, brave and hard-living." In short, the author
suggests that the very behaviors men are socialized to perform
are, in large part, directly contributing to the sex
differential in mortality. Cultural and behavioral changes are
recommended as a possible method of decreased male mortality.
Waldron's review of the literature also points to a recent
decrease in the gap between male and female mortality (a trend
not seen in suicide, see John McIntosh & Barb Jewell, 1986,
Suicide and Life-Threatening Behavior, 16(1)); she predicts
that as women incorporate more of the traditionally male
life-threatening behaviors in to their lifestyles (i.e.,
smoking, drinking, motor vehicle accidents often related to
drinking), the mortality gap may continue to decrease. The
cultural and behavioral changes Waldon recommends would be
beneficial to men (in reducing mortality rates) and to women as
well (in allowing them to succeed vocationally without the
elevated mortality rates currently suffered by men).

3-065   Weiss, James   M. A. (1968).   Suicide   in   the   aged.   In
        H. L. P. Resnik   (Ed.),   Suicidal   behaviors: Diagnosis   and
        management (pp. 255–267).   Boston: Little, Brown.

        The author reviews various demographic factors in suicide.   The
        correlation of suicide rates with age is discussed along with
        the lack of empirical literature in this area.   Diagnostic
        considerations in predicting suicide potential are listed (older
        persons, males, divorced or separated persons, socially isolated
        persons, previous history of suicide attempts, etc.).   Data from
        a World Health Organization report is cited as evidence that
        while general suicide rates in males have decreased over the
        past few decades, the suicide rates of elderly males now
        comprise a greater proportion of suicides than ever before.
        Conversely, suicide rates among women have been increasing, due
        to both a proportionate and absolute increase in the rates for
        older females.   Weiss also describes factors other than age
        which affect suicide rates in the general population.   Older
        persons tend to use the same methods for successful suicide as
        the general population, although there is some preference for
        more violent and efficient methods (see also McIntosh & Santos,
        1985–86, reference 4–063).   Older persons are seen as more
        serious in their suicidal attempts, and as less likely to use
        suicidal gestures in a manipulative attempt for attention.
        Durkheim's (reference 3–014) concept of anomie and the
        psychoanalytic identification of suicide with self-directed
        aggressive tendencies are discussed.   Indicators of suicide
        potential (aging, loss, psychiatric disorder), warning signs
        (withdrawal, rejection of loved ones, suicide threats, making
        out a will under unusual circumstances), and implications for
        prevention and treatment are presented.   Weiss focuses on
        depression and/or psychiatric disorders coupled with increasing
        age. He concludes that suicidal behavior among the old is most
        often a symptom of cultural, psychological, or biological
        disorder, not a free moral choice.   Basic scientists, behavioral
        investigators, public health specialists, social activists, and
        clinicians are encouraged to work together for prediction,
        prevention, and treatment of suicidal behavior among the aged.

3-066   Wiendieck, G. (1970).   Social determinants of suicide in old
        age. In   Richard   Fox   (Ed.),   Proceedings: Fifth international
        conference for suicide prevention, London, September 24–27, 1969
        (pp. 196–197).   Vienna: International Association for Suicide
        Prevention.

        The author focuses on the sociogenic variables found in most
        civilized countries of the world that are responsible for the
        high suicide rates of the old. The lack of meaningful social
        roles for the old is cited as one such factor.   In addition, old
        age creates a variety of conflicts which require adjustment or,
        if adjustment is not adequate, may result in suicide.   The
        problem of trying to ascertain reliable information about the
        causes of suicide when the victim is dead is mentioned.   A study
        is discussed which considered the latent predispositions to

suicide. It was observed that many older people (mean age=73) expressed resignation and a tiredness of life. Another study revealed lower levels of life satisfaction in older people with suicidal thoughts. Individuals with suicidal ideation also felt lonely more often, had trouble making contacts with others, and were more often negative.

CASE STUDIES

3-067 Alleged attempt at suicide by a woman of seventy-one who stated that she had grown desperate regarding her economic situation: Discussion of the mental state. (1929-1931).   International Clinics, 3(Series 40-5), 64-67.

A case study is presented of a woman, aged 71, who attempted suicide by laudanum overdose. She explained to hospital staff that she wished to end her life because she had no money for food and clothing and no charitable organization would agree to help her. Her affective state (i.e., cheerful, contented) is described and a tentative diagnosis of manic-depressive constitution is suggested. The woman was discharged after negotations with social services for assistance.

3-068 Haggerty, Judith. (1973). Suicide in the aging: Suicidal behavior in a 70-year-old man: A case report. Journal of Geriatric Psychiatry, 6, 43-51.

Haggerty, a psychiatric social worker, provides a detailed case study of a 70-year-old widower who made three suicide attempts within a four month period prior to his admission to a hospital. His wife had died from cancer just over one year prior to the admission. Mr. Jorgenson, the widower, had a stable work history, working for the same company from his late 20s until his retirement. At the time of the hospitalization he lived in an apartment in the downstairs of one of his daughter's homes. His son-in-law and three preschool children lived in the home as well. Mr. Jorgenson was very dependent on his wife when she was alive. He had a long history of physical health problems ranging from blood disorders, vascular problems, to rheumatiod arthritis. The latter caused increasing disability and resulted in the move of he and his wife into the apartment in their daughter's home three years earlier.   The home was in Massachusetts and he had lived in New York. The medical problems worsened after the wife's death and he was hospitalized on several occasions. Mr. Jorgenson suffered periodically over his life from depression. He often talked about death and suicide, had stated his philosophical acceptance of suicide as a reasonable coping mechanism for problems. He had also stated that he did not wish to live past the age of 70. Following his wife's death, Mr. Jorgenson had displayed depression, withdrawal from activities he had previously enjoyed, insomnia, weight loss, fatigue, increasing isolation in his own apartment, and had told his internist that "life was no longer worth living." Sleeping pills had been prescribed for the insomnia and were the method employed in both of the first two attempts. In midwinter he was missed and discovered by his daughter a few hours after taking the pills and remained comatose for three days. Upon recovery he was released with no psychiatric treatment or referral. His daughter took control of and carefully released to him his sleeping pills thereafter. His depression continued at severe levels and in early spring, close to the anniversary of his wife's death and just days before his own 70th birthday, he again took an overdose of sleeping pills that he was able to obtain when the daughter was out of the house. He was comatose for 24 hours and upon recovery was released again, but this time a referral was made to a psychiatrist who prescribed antidepressant medication and outpatient therapy. Less than two weeks later Mr. Jorgenson came to his daughter and admitted to her that he had again attempted suicide, this time by drinking a caustic cleaning agent. Rather than dying however, he simply vomited and now could barely swallow anything because of the burns in his mouth and throat. At this time the psychiatrist referred him for hospitalization. Antidepressants, activities, interpersonal contacts, and therapies were provided during the hospitalization and when it was deemed appropriate he was discharged. Following an incident in which he bled from a cut to his leg he was again hospitalized although he insisted that he had not done it intentionally or with the intent to commit suicide. At this point his daughter was unwilling to have him return to her home and following his release he agreed to enter a residential home. At the time of this article he had been living in the home for eight months and seemed to be active and adjusting well with only occasional depression. The case is further discussed by a number of professionals in the same issue of this journal (see reference 3–019).

3–069   Hickman, Jack W. (1965). Attempted suicide in the aged. Journal of the Indiana State Medical Association, 58, 1138–1140.

Following the more detailed presentation of one case of an elderly suicide attempter and three brief additional cases, Hickman briefly discusses the literature on suicide attempts and the high risk elderly for attempts. The case presented in detail involved a 90-year-old white male brought to a general hospital following the discovery of him in his garage with the lawn mower running and the doors closed. His wife made the discovery, pulled him out of the garage, and called police for help. His health was generally good, although he had undergone successful surgery for carcinoma of the larynx six years before the attempt. He had experienced failing vision due to cataracts in recent months and had become somewhat depressed as a result because he worried he would become a burden for his wife. The couple's financial circumstances were generally good. He had left a suicide note explaining he had not wanted to become a burden and asking for forgiveness. He was fully alert four hours after admission and was willing to talk about his suicide attempt. Psychiatric consultation revealed no organic brain syndromes or psychotic disorders. The availability of surgery for his cataracts was explained to him and this produced elevation of mood and eager consent to the surgery. Following the successful surgery the patient was much improved with apparently no depression or suicide ideation.

3–070 McIntosh, John L., Hubbard, Richard W., & Santos, John F. (1981). Suicide among the elderly: A review of issues with case studies. Journal of Gerontological Social Work, 4, 63–74.

This article reviews the literature on elderly suicide levels, motivations, and prevention. In addition two cases taken from those of an outreach program that serves the frail and vulnerable elderly are presented. Of the first 200 clients of this program during an 18 month period, 16% displayed suicidal behavior ranging from statements of intent to recent attempts.

The first case involved a 76-year-old male who after receiving a diagnosis of operable cancer refused the surgery and stated that "When the pain gets real bad, I'll take care of things myself." The physician notified the outreach program and a home visit was arranged that same day. The man's wife had died two years before from the same type of cancer he now had and her surgery had only prolonged her pain. He stated that he had lived his life and he was now ready to die. He had no history of mental illness or suicide attempts. He died 10 months later. This case could be classified as an example of indirect self-destructive behavior in which the omission of the surgery resulted in death sooner than might have been expected with the surgery. This example of a "rational suicide" poses a difficult dilemma for caseworkers.

The second case involved a 67-year-old woman who had a history of chronic depression, alcoholism, and suicide attempts in middle age. At age 64 she had made two additional attempts, one shortly after the death of her husband and the other four months later. After the second attempt she was institutionalized and referred to the outreach program. After her discharge she received weekly visits by caseworkers and was seeing a psychiatrist. Her son moved far away from her six weeks after her discharge and she threatened suicide again which resulted in a short-term institutionalization. This woman's history of attempts as well as her alcoholism and depressive history, coupled with the recent losses allowed early identification as a potential risk for suicide. Contact with the psychiatrist and frequent visitations and other referrals were therefore able to be employed to deal with circumstances as they occurred.

3–071 Miller, Marv. (1977). A psychological autopsy of a geriatric suicide. Journal of Geriatric Psychiatry, 10, 229–242.

Miller describes an intensive case study (a "psychological autopsy") for an elderly male who committed suicide and was part of the sample he studied in Arizona (see Miller, 1978b, reference 4–066). Miller was asked to conduct the careful study by the daughter of the deceased who was having difficulty dealing with her father's death because she felt she needed an answer to the question "Why?". The father had been a widower for over three years at his death and had retired in April and committed suicide in November of the same year. The deceased lived with his single daughter who was in her 30s. During the period after his retirement he kept himself busy primarily by raising bees and selling the honey. In June of the year he died and retired, he returned to his Alabama hometown, dated the widow of a childhood friend, and they decided to get married. The fiance's job forced her to remain in Alabama until her pension eligibility was reached in two years. After a stay in Alabama the father returned to Arizona and his daughter. During October friends began to notice that he was depressed. During conversations with a sister and in several other subtle ways, the man gave warning signs to his suicide that were apparently not recognized as such until after his death. He expressed regret that he had retired and shortly thereafter his former employer contacted him and asked him to return to work on a full-time basis to help them out in their busy season. He was to return to work on the following Monday. He had stated his concern over financial matters and his need to support his daughter and fiance. The job would provide an opportunity to resolve those concerns, or so it would seem. There were indications of stress and insomnia on his part but he also spoke of future plans, particularly to his fiance two days before he killed himself (Friday). He also remarked in that telephone conversation that he was "so tired." On Saturday he insisted that his daughter prepare a grocery list so that he could go shopping and the daughter suspected, in hindsight, that what he actually wanted was an excuse to go out so that he could buy shotgun shells. Later on Saturday he checked his papers and insurance policies. On Sunday, the day of his suicide, he drove his daughter to church but claimed that he felt too bad to attend himself. He returned home, went to his den and killed himself with a shotgun blast to his chest. His daughter returned home from church to discover his body. Miller analyzes the case and suggests that the depression that the father was displaying was far too great to be explained solely by his recent, self-chosen early retirement and his plans for a future wedding seem to lessen the likelihood that the loss of his wife over three years earlier was a major factor. He killed himself on the day before he was to return to work and Miller feels that his statement of "I am so tired" might be an important one. It is conjectured that the man was "psychologically exhausted," facing what seems to be a distored perception of his financial problems. He had worked hard all his life, had chosen to retire early, and now he was going back to work in order to once again make money to support others. Miller feels that the illogical nature of the suicidal mind may have produced the distorted financial impression he had. One of Miller's concluding remarks is that the father had several potential factors that may have produced suicidal feelings "and each in its own way appears to have diminished the quality of life as only he could have

defined that quality" (p. 240).   According to Miller, the man
perceived himself to have few if any options.   This case also
appears in Miller (1979, reference 3-027) on pages 82-90.

3-072 Minden, Sarah L. (1984).   Elderly psychiatric   emergency
patients.   In E. L. Bassuk & A. W. Birk (Eds.), Emergency
psychiatry: Concepts, methods, practices (pp. 351-369,
especially pp. 365-366, "Suicide"). New York: Plenum Press.

This chapter was written for emergency setting personnel and
includes a brief case example of an elderly suicide that
presented to such personnel but was not acted upon.   An
81-year-old male was the deceased and his suicide followed his
wife's death from a sudden heart attack four months before. The
man had not cried at the funeral and in the period afterward he
isolated himself in the house and neglected eating and going to
bed except when a housekeeper forced him to do so. He sat in a
chair and stared blankly. He was hospitalized for pneumonia and
recovered after a hospital stay of one week. He talked repeated
about death and his son took him to the emergency room where the
emergency personnel simply told them that it would take time for
him to recover from his wife's death. He was offered sleeping
pills to help him sleep. Three days later, after updating his
will, putting his affairs in order, and leaving a note, he
hanged himself in his garage by his belt. Minden suggests that
the circumstances and signs that he had been giving should have
prompted action by the emergency personnel due to their
indication of suicidal risk.

3-073 Moriwaki, Sharon Y. (1981).   Ethnicity and aging.   In Irene
M. Burnside (Ed.), Nursing and the aged (2nd ed.) (pp. 612-629,
especially p. 612). New York: McGraw-Hill.

This chapter on aging and ethnicity begins with a case example
of a 71-year-old Japanese-American man's suicide. He had spent
10 years caring for his wife during her physical decline until
she died less than a year before. He now felt alone although he
lived with his oldest son and family and his other children and
their families visited often. He began to show a lessening of
interest in usually enjoyable activities (reading the Japanese
newspaper, fishing) and despaired over his own physical
complaints. He felt he would not get well and may become a
burden as his wife had been in her illness.   Shortly after a
hospitalization and surgery he hanged himself in the son's
garage. Moriwaki interpreted the case and emphasized the
socialization of the deceased, his lack of status in his old
age, his lack of achievement and acculturation to U.S. society,
his feelings that he did not contribute to his son's family and
may become a burden.   Under these circumstances, and
understanding the situation as it would be for one of his
ethnicity, the circumstances were unbearable and "he took the
acceptable Japanese strategy of coping" (p. 615) by killing
himself. Moriwaki's point in the case is that in order to
understand elderly members of ethnic minorities, we must

understand the values, expectations, past history, and personal circumstances.

3-074   Neale, John M., Oltmanns, Thomas F., & Davison, Gerald C. (1982). Case studies in abnormal psychology (pp. 279-295, "Depression and a suicidal attempt in an older adult"). New York: Wiley.

In this chapter the authors present a case study of Helen Kay, age 73, who attempted to commit suicide by drinking herself into a stupor and then walking out into the ocean to drown. Police found Mrs. Kay lying on the pier, bottle in hand. She had gotten so drunk that she passed out before attempting to drown herself. When police found her, she was in a delerious state, confused and frightened, and she was nearly frozen. Relating her recent and past history, the authors discuss Mrs. Kay's recent episodes of heavy drinking, her sad, despondent moods, and her recent physical complaints and verbal abuse of other residents in her retirement hotel. They also describe a past history of episodes of depression in college and throughout her adult life, as well as Mrs. Kay's feeling that she was/is responsible for what happens to her husband and children. Mrs. Kay suffered several major losses. Her husband died of lung cancer and also suffered from senile dementia. Mrs. Kay felt responsible for his death. Afterward, she sold her home and moved into the retirement home, another loss.

Mrs. Kay, upon the urging of her son, entered a program of cognitive therapy to help her find other solutions to her problems and deal with her depression. After 30 therapy sessions Mrs. Kay felt less responsibility for her husband's death, was happier than she had been in a long time, and successfully quit drinking. The case demonstrates some of the personal factors related to suicidal behavior in the elderly, as well as the positive benefits of therapy for suicidal elderly individuals.

3-075   Niswander, G. Donald, Casey, Thomas M., & Humphrey, John A. (1973). A panorama of suicide: A casebook of psychological autopsies (pp. 117-125, "Elderly sick suicide"). Springfield, IL: Thomas.

The cases of two elderly female suicides (one aged 67, the other aged 85) are presented. Both women had fairly normal early life histories. Both had careers and had been fairly independent all of their lives. Both suffered a debilitating illness in the later stage of life which left them dependent and depressed and unable to pursue their former life style. One of the two committed suicide by drowning while the other took an overdose of sleeping pills. In each case relatives and/or physicians were aware of the negative emotional state of the individual, but they did nothing to prevent the suicide. [From the standpoint of typical cases, these two are atypical since the most likely elderly suicide is a male who uses a lethal method.]

Case examples of elderly suicide and suicide attempts may be found also in the following references: 3-002, 3-008, 3-011, 3-017, 3-027, 3-032, 3-034, 3-058,   3-076,   3-077, 3-078, 3-081, 3-082, 4-012, 4-022, 4-023, 4-052, 5-047, 5-079, 5-085.

ETHICS AND ELDERLY SUICIDE

3-076 Bromberg, Shirley, & Cassel, Christine K. (1983).   Suicide in the elderly: The limits of paternalism.   Journal of the American Geriatrics Society, 31, 698-703.

The authors begin their article with a case report of an 84-year-old man who attempted suicide four months after his wife of 50 years died.   The attempt was made by slashing both wrists with a razor blade.   Following treatment for his wounds as well as psychiatric and antidepressant treatment, the staff and especially the family felt the man was still suicidal.   He was hospitalized until the staff felt the risk was gone and he demanded to be released.   His family persisted in their wish to have him remain hospitalized.   He was nonetheless discharged and several months later was living at home apparently without depressive symptomatology.

The main focus of this article is on paternalism with respect to care for the elderly.   The authors feel that caregivers of the old at times are overly paternalistic and their actions are not always in the best interest of the patient.   They advocate treatment which respects the autonomy of the individual.   The authors briefly discuss suicide, bereavement, social and religious beliefs and attitudes toward suicide in the old, and medical considerations.   For the latter, they present the work of Szasz (see e.g., reference 3-084) who maintains that suicidal thoughts are not symptoms of a mental illness and therefore do not warrant coercion with respect to treatment.   Intervention may in fact represent interference with individual liberty.   The authors suggest that the rights of the individual to self-determination must be maintained although in the case of depression, confusion, or other mental disorder, there is a need for intervention because the person cannot decide for themselves.   They recommend that the autonomy of the individual be protected and considered with respect as the key issue or concern.   Paternalism should be carefully applied and only when truly necessary.

3-077 Lesnoff-Caravaglia, Gari. (1980, November).   Suicide in old age: An ethical dilemma.   Paper presented at the 33rd annual meeting of the Gerontological Society of America, San Diego.

This paper begins with three clinical vignettes of elderly suicides.   Life expectancy increases have led us to consider self-determined death as a possibility.   The author portrays aged suicide as being motivated by an interest in "closing life with meaning, rather than despairing at the meaninglessness of life" (p. 3). The person wishes an end to life and a peace. The author feels that the old are free to choose suicide and are solely responsible for their own lives. She claims that in modern technological society the old moral/philosophical views and condemnations of suicide are no longer valid (they are an anachronism). Life is different in this era and suicide ("self-determination") must be considered in that light. The individual, their circumstances and beliefs about life must be understood with respect to the morality of their choice. The paper concludes with recommendations for practitioners with the above viewpoint as the starting point for those recommendations.

3-078 Moody, H. R. (1984). Can suicide on grounds of old age be ethically justified? In Margot Tallmer, Elizabeth R. Prichard, Austin H. Kutscher, Robert DeBellis, Mahlon S. Hale, & Ivan K. Goldberg (Eds.), The life-threatened elderly (pp. 64-92). New York: Columbia University Press.

According to Moody, elderly suicide takes on importance at this time at unprecedented levels because life expectancy has increased and the tremendous rate of cultural change has lessened the importance of the old and the roles they play, thus lessening the things that "make life worth living" (p. 64). Moody wants to consider whether suicide on the grounds of old age can be ethically justified. Moody first suggests that suicide can be a "rational" choice in such a way that a person can make a life choice after considered deliberation in which the choice can be made either to commit suicide or not do so. Three points of view that weaken the possibility of ethically justifying suicide in old age are briefly considered: the sanctity-of-life, libertarian, and view that suicide is a form of mental illness arguments. Moody next turns his attention to the ideology of suicide prevention, that is, life is good and it is better to live than die. However, he suggests this is not a good argument against elderly suicide, nor is our duty to others or duty to self arguments that are often made. In the case of the old we have an individual who is making a deliberate, non-impulsive choice of suicide, who has a negative outlook for the future, has disengaged from society and society from him/her, and who is at the end of their natural lifespan so that the death is not "premature." Moody next considers the argument for suicide in old age, proceeding through the "balance sheet" and quality-of-life arguments. Brief case examples of each are given. The final conclusion is that neither of these arguments are fundamentally sound and compelling to justify suicide on the grounds of old age either. The arguments for suicide on the grounds of old age are essentially stating that old age is meaningless and not worth living. Moody argues that at any age, even to one's last breath, new goals are possible that can give old age meaning. The author worries not that Nazi-like "legally enforced euthanasia" will develop, but rather that moral attitudes will change, what Moody called "a climate of opinion," such that "avoidance of suicide [might be seen] as a matter of

shame or cowardice--selfishly being a 'burden on society'"
(p. 89). Suicide under these circumstances becomes a moral
obligation, not a right (or choice) but rather a duty. It is
because of this possible "slippery slope" that Moody feels we as
a society must look and find new meaning in old age.

3-079 Portwood, Doris. (1978). Common-sense suicide: The final
       right. New York: Dodd, Mead. [An excerpt appears under the
       title "A right to suicide?" in Psychology Today, January 1978,
       pp. 66, 68, 71, 73-74, 76]

Portwood, herself a "senior citizen," argues that suicide is a
right of the elderly. This is contended because society permits
nor provides any "good death" for its citizens who have
rationally decided that they wish to die. Portwood does not
argue for suicide as a right at any age, rather presenting her
points for the later period of life with its relentless losses
and negative aspects. A major component of Portwood's case
revolves around the concept of "balance sheet suicide," where an
elderly person can rationally weigh the positive forces and
circumstances in their life against the negative ones and if
they feel the negative outweigh the positive, choose suicide.
Her goal is to make such a rational choice of death legally
sanctioned. She argues not to eliminate old age or the aged,
but rather to allow a right to die, which she feels implies also
the right to life among those who do not choose self-determined
death.

3-080 Pressey, Sidney L. (1977). Comment: Any rights as to my dying?
       Gerontologist, 17, 296, 302.

Pressey discusses his internship experiences with attempting to
measure mental deterioration in the elderly and subsequent
professional endeavors. Now, at 88, he expresses concerns with
the connotations of suicide in our society, and the lack of
individual choice in dying. Pressey expresses concern about the
plight of the old, with no one to turn to in order to facilitate
death. He urges legislation to protect the right to die, rather
than legislation which inflicts inhumane suffering for the
extension of life, and advocates national attention focused on
the best ways to serve the very old and their families.

3-081 Pretzel, Paul W. (1968). Philosophical and ethical
       considerations of suicide prevention. Bulletin of Suicidology,
       No. 7, 30-38. (Reprinted in Brent Q. Hafen & Eugene J. Faux
       (Eds.) (1971), Self-destructive behavior: A national crisis
       (pp. 269-284). Minneapolis, MN: Burgess. Reprinted in Robert
       F. Weir (Ed.) (1977), Ethical issues in death and dying
       (pp. 387-400). New York: Columbia University Press.)

Pretzel describes the polarity between individual freedom and
social cohesion as a philosophical question encompassing such
diverse areas as birth control, capital punishment, abortion,
euthanasia, suicide, and suicide prevention. The right to kill

oneself has been debated since earliest records of Greek philosophy. Plato, Socrates, the Epicureans, Stoics, and philosophers of the Enlightenment, all endorsed the right to commit suicide given appropriate circumstances (i.e., generally, we have the right to choose, but the choice should be made from courage, not as an escape). Not all philosophers have endorsed the right to kill oneself. Pythagoras, Aristotle, Kant, Schopenhauer, and William James described suicide as a rebellion against the gods, a cowardly act, inconsistent with the categorical imperative, ambivalent cries for help, and a denial of the task to find religious meaning, respectively. Judaic and Christian religions offer similar sanctions against suicide. Contemporary society often endorses four types of suicide as being "rational": (1) suicide for the good of a cause (e.g., military heroism), (2) suicide as a reaction to a painful debilitating situation (e.g., lingering terminal illness), (3) situations in which a person is no longer gaining pleasure from life, and (4) love-pact suicides. Case illustrations are presented to depict each of the types. Suicide which stems from an apparently hopeless situation is considered rational. The prototype is an elderly person suffering from a chronic, painful, terminal illness. The major question for the clinician or other person confronted with a suicidal situation is when, if ever, one is willing to say "Yes, I agree. It is the best thing for you to do, and I have no right to interfere, so I won't."

3-082   Rollin, Betty. (1985). <u>Last wish</u>. New York: Linden Press/Simon and Schuster.

Rollin's book describes her experience with her 76-year-old mother who committed suicide with the indirect aid of Rollin. The mother was diagnosed with ovarian cancer in 1981 and committed suicide in 1983. This book chronicles the events of this time period and the steps that culminated in the self-chosen death. Rollin's mother was in great pain and pain-killing medications had become ineffective. Chemotherapy and its side-effects had taken a toll as well. The mother had been given six months to live when she asked her daughter to help her to die/kill herself. Rollin contacted many U.S. physicians in what proved to be a futile attempt to discover a combination of drugs that would provide a swift and painless suicide. This information was however provided by an Amsterdam physician. Rollin acquired the drugs for her mother, who was given the drugs and then took them in the presence of Rollin. Rollin presents her mother's suicide as a rational choice to end a life that had only a negative outlook. Death offered her mother "a door" through which she passed and ended a painful existence.

3-083   Saul, Shura, & Saul, Sidney R. (1977). Old people talk about--The right to die. <u>Omega</u>, <u>8</u>, 129-139.

A dialogue-form discussion is presented among eight members of an HRF (Health Related Facility) regarding the right to live or

die. The members disagreed philosophically on the issue of
suicide and were unwilling to compromise their positions. The
expression of emotions and opinions surrounding the right to
live or die seemed to promote enthusiasm for life among all
group members.

3-084   Szasz, Thomas S. (1971). The ethics of suicide. The Antioch
Review, 31, 7-17.

Szasz denounces the traditional view of suicide as a
manifestation of pathology and distinguishes between three often
confused categories of suicide: suicide proper (successful
suicide), attempted or threatened suicide (unsuccessful
suicide), and attribution of suicidal intent to another
individual. Szasz emphasizes that the first two categories
refer to acts by actual or supposedly suicidal persons, while
the third refers to the claim of an ostensibly normal person
about someone else's suicidal ideations. He believes successful
suicide is radically different from unsuccessful suicide (i.e.,
successful suicide is committed by a person who intends to die
while unsuccessful attempts are made by persons attempting to
change their lives, not terminate them) and thus, the two
categories should not be discussed simultaneously. He focuses,
in this article, on suicide proper.

Szasz criticizes the mental health tradition of taking control
of a suicidal person's situation (does confiding suicidal
thoughts deprive the patient of the basic human freedom to grant
or withold consent for treatment?). Traditional psychiatric
belief on suicide intervention springs from the concept of
mental illness as the root of suicidal behavior. Szasz concedes
that suicidal behavior may be "exceedingly disturbing" for
significant persons in the suicidal "patient's" life. However,
he rejects the conclusion that the suicidal person is disturbed
and therefore mentally ill and requiring psychiatric
hospitalization and treatment. If the person is troubled by
suicidal inclinations, treatment is generally desirable, but in
situations where physicians and psychiatrists intervene without
the patient's permission, treatment is unconscionable. Szasz
hypothesizes that suicidal persons challenge the basic values of
physicians. Physicians therefore feel the need (perhaps
unconsciously) to save the suicidal person from themselves (or
perhaps, to save the physician or psychiatrist from confronting
their own doubts about the value of life). Suicide is medical
heresy. Szasz argues that psychiatric methods of suicide
prevention often aggravate rather than relieve the suicidal
person's distress, and consequently, increase the desire for
self-destruction. He describes "deceptive" practices used by
suicide prevention centers to keep intently suicidal persons
from committing "self-murder." Suicide prevention is
conceptualized as a "political act on the person." Essentially,
if suicide is an expression of human freedom, prevention can
only succeed by curtailing freedom; deprivation of liberty
becomes a psychiatric treatment.

4
EMPIRICAL INVESTIGATIONS: ANNOTATIONS

4-001   Abel, Ernest L., & Zeidenberg, Phillip. (1985).   Age, alcohol
and violent death: A postmortem study.   Journal of Studies on
Alcohol, 46, 228-231.

This investigation presents data gleaned from a retrospective
analysis of chief medical examiner's records for Erie County, NY
(which includes Buffalo) from 1973 through 1983.   Data are
considered only for violent causes of death (traffic accidents,
miscellaneous accidents, homicide, suicide).   From among a total
of 6036 deaths during the period of study, 3374 were
violence-related and blood alcohol levels (BAL) were available
for 3358.   Suicides represented 20.5% of the 3358 deaths.   The
available records included chromatography results to indicate
BAL.   Alcohol involvement was defined as BALs equal to or above
10 mg/dl and intoxication was defined as equal to or above 100
mg/dl.   By these criteria, a total of 42.5% of violent death
victims had been drinking prior to death and 31.4% had been
intoxicated (74% of the alcohol involved;   compared to only
15.6% and 7.2% of natural deaths, drinking and intoxicated,
respectively).   Drinking prior to death was found in 35.4% of
the suicides, while intoxication was seen in 22.8% (both figures
the lowest among violent death categories).   Men, blacks, and
the young (especially 14-24) had the highest rates of alcohol
involvement among victims of violent death.   Those 75 years of
age and above had the lowest percentage of victims drinking
prior to death.   Among all age groupings, including 64-74 and
75+, there were more nonalcohol-related than alcohol-related
suicides (the figures for those 64-74 were approximately 11-12%
vs. 4-5%, respectively).   From this study it is implied that
alcohol and/or intoxication is involved in fewer violent deaths
for the old than those of other ages.   Exact comparisons among
age groups are not possible, however, because virtually no
specific data (numbers, percentages, or rates) are given for the
elderly age groups (64-74 and 75+).

4-002   Abrahams, Ruby R., & Patterson, Robert D. (1978-79).
Psychological distress among the community elderly: Prevalence,
characteristics and implications for service.   International

Journal of Aging and Human Development, 9, 1-18.

This article reports the results of a survey of 445 elderly
individuals (64-74 and 75+) from a predominantly white, middle
class New England town. The sample was drawn from town census
lists with a 23% refusal rate. The authors argue convincingly
that the sample selection is likely to yield conservative (i.e.,
low) estimates of the levels of psychological distress among
these community-dwelling elderly. Social workers interviewed
the participants (and in about half the cases, with other family
members present and contributing) regarding five self-reported
indicators of psychological impairment (depression, current
mental health problems, periods of inability to function due to
emotional upset, suicidal ideation, alcohol problems). A total
of 8% of the sample indicated feelings of depression "all the
time" or "everyday"; 4% volunteered information regarding
current psychiatric problems; 3% had experienced worry,
nervousness, or emotional upset that kept them from carrying on
usual activities for two weeks or more within the past three
years; 2% (N=9) said they had experienced suicidal thoughts;
and 2% admitted to current alcohol problems. The
suicide-related questions produced great anxiety on the part of
many respondents and the authors suggest that the 2% figure is
especially suspect. Some respondents became agitated when asked
about suicidal thoughts; two stopped the interview and refused
to go on; three more would answer no more suicide-related
questions. There were 20 respondents who admitted and willingly
discussed suicidal ideation at some time in their lives. Of
these, 65% had had these thoughts since the age of 60.
Combining all measures, 17% of the current sample showed one or
more indicators of psychological impairment. No age or sex
differences in psychological impairment were found, but impaired
elderly: more frequently lived in deteriorated neighborhoods,
had lower levels of education, more often had physical
impairments, were being cared for by spouse or family, were
unable to develop relationships beyond their household, and more
often had a past history of psychopathology. Although these
life-interfering impairments would indicate a need for mental
health services, almost none of these elderly had utilized such
services (either the healthy or unhealthy respondents), they
were largely unaware of the services in their community, and
were reluctant to use them if they knew of them. The authors
suggest increased community support systems, lessening of the
difficulty to utilize effectively the existing mental health
services, and community mental health education to prevent and
lessen such problems among the elderly.

4-003   Ahlburg, Dennis A., & Schapiro, Morton O. (1984). Socioeconomic
ramifications of changing cohort size: An analysis of
U.S. postwar suicide rates by age and sex. Demography, 21,
97-108.

These authors apply a "relative cohort size model" theory to the
understanding of suicide rates. They suggest that the size of

cohorts (groups of people born in the same period of time), relative to the size of other cohorts in the population had direct economic and indirect social impact on suicide rates (one measure of stress). This paper first explains the involved theory (model) as it would apply to suicide among the young (14-44) and "older" (45-64) cohorts. The ratio of younger (16-29) to older (30-64) males was used as the measure of relative cohort size (RCS). This model was then tested by looking at the relation between the RCS measure and suicide rates (1948-1976) for younger and older males and females. Decreases in the RCS ratio (fewer young compared to older males) was expected to be associated with lessened suicide rates for the young because young males would have a better employment experience and incomes closer to their expectations and needs when there are fewer of them competing for jobs. Young females would also experience lower rates because of increased household income and indirectly by lessened stress leading to perhaps fewer divorces as well (this rationale is tied very much to the non-career woman who works in the home predominantly if not exclusively). Another result of greater household income would be that fewer young females would likely enter the labor force and therefore competition for jobs will lessen for older females. Therefore, the suicide rates for older females should also decline. For older males, however, decreases in this ratio leads to worsening labor market position relative to the income aspirations and thus increased suicide rates. Increases in the RCS ratio, on the other hand, would directly affect employment experiences and relative income and indirectly affect labor force participation and other factors such as divorce so that rates of suicide for the young of both sexes and older females would increase while those for older males would decrease. From the standpoint of prediction and explanation of past trends, the authors suggest that the latter (ratio increases) reflect the post-war rates to the present (1976), while in the future demographic changes are expected to produce the former (decreased RCS levels). Therefore, as the large "baby boomer" cohort ages, relatively good economic circumstances for the young are anticipated as well as a reversal in suicide rates for those under 35. However, at the same time, a worsening relative economic position should lead to increased suicide rates for the over 45 age groups. "Therefore, the problem group in terms of suicide during this and the next decade will be older men, rather than younger men and women as it was in the 1960s and 1970s" (p. 103). The authors suggest that to combat these trends policy needs to be directed to improve the labor market experience for these older males and decrease the unemployment rates. While this article is directed more at the "middle aged" (44-64) age groups than those over 65, some of the same arguments for older males in particular could be made with regard to those who remain in the labor force and those who may feel pressured to leave the labor force before they wish to do so as there are larger numbers of middle aged males competing for jobs.

4-004   Atchley, Robert C. (1980). Aging and suicide: Reflections   on
the quality   of   life?   In Suzanne G. Haynes & Manning Feinleib
(Eds.), Second   conference   on   the   epidemiology   of   aging
(pp. 141–158;   Discussion, pp. 158–161).   Washington,   D.C.:
United States   Government   Printing   Office.   NIH   Publication
No. 80–969.

Atchley considers three sets of data to determine the effects of
age on suicide and particularly suicide in the aged. The first
set of data consists of cross-national suicide figures published
by the World Health Organization for 20   nations   from   1955 to
1966 by age and sex. The second set of data is official suicide
figures published   by   the   United   States'   National Center for
Health Statistics for the time period 1955 to 1968.   The   final
set consists of a cohort analysis of age-specific data for the
U.S. for the years 1920 to 1965 (males only included).   The
cross-national data reveal a nearly universal, high positive
correlation between age and suicide rates for males.   Atchley
states that "Culture thus appears to have an impact on the level
of reported   suicide   among   males within various countries, but
very little impact on the age trend" (p. 143).   Much less
consistent correlations are observed for females and age. Male
rates were observed to be higher than those for females at all
ages   and   in   all   countries.   Stepwise multiple regression
analysis was performed for 10 chronic disease death rates by age
and their influence on suicide rates. After age 65, but not for
the age groups from 45 to 64, the death rates for these chronic
diseases produces a high multiple R for both sexes. These
latter results do not indicate that the presence of chronic
disease will cause suicide among an individual. Instead, they
indicate that in cultures where there are high suicide rates
there are also high chronic disease death rates, especially
after age 65.

The U.S. data showed the increase in youth suicide rates and the
declines in rates for the old.   Atchley notes however that
neither retirement nor the empty nest syndrome seem to influence
the suicide rates of males and females, respectively, in any
significant fashion. He bases this on the fact that no surge is
seen in rates immediately after retirement age for men, nor for
the ages 45–54 for females. The cohort analysis data considered
show historical periods' differential influences on suicide
rates and, different from studies with more contemporary cohorts
(e.g., Solomon & Murphy, 1984, reference 4–095), "what appears
to be a leveling off of suicide rates for the younger cohorts
since 1955" (p. 154) was observed. A number of excellent tables
and figures displaying the data of the study are presented.
Atchley concludes his paper with the implications of his
findings. He suggests that the technique of psychological
autopsies needs to be employed more often, that
multidisciplinary and multicausal methods and theories need to
be employed to study and explain suicidal behavior, and that
estimates of "true" levels of active and passive suicide are
needed. A discussion of Atchley's paper appears also.

4-005   Atkinson, Maxwell. (1971). The Samaritans and the elderly: Some problems in communication between a suicide prevention scheme and a group with a high suicide rate. Social Sciences and Medicine, 5, 483-490. [Essentially the same article appears as "The Samaritans and the elderly: Problems of communication," in Richard Fox (Ed.). (1970), Proceedings of the fifth international conference for suicide prevention (London, September 24-27, 1969) (pp. 159-166). Vienna: International Association for Suicide Prevention.]

The study results related in this paper give some information about the underrepresentativeness of the old in the caseloads of suicide prevention and crisis intervention services using telephones as the primary contact mode. The results were part of a larger study in Britain of communication and its relationship to isolation. In the fall of 1968 a national random survey of those over age 65 was conducted by a market research agency employing a questionnaire designed by Atkinson. A response rate of 75% was realized, representing 583 completed interviews. The questionnaire asked about telephone usage, social contacts and isolation, and included four questions about the Samaritans, the primary suicide prevention scheme in Britain (there are chapters of the Samaritans worldwide but it began in Britain). The questions about the Samaritans are the focus of this report. A total of 41% of these elderly individuals said they had heard of the Samaritan organization, but only 28% could actually tell what the organization did. Knowledge of the Samaritans was defined as being able to know what the agency did. The other two questions asked if the individual knew the name of their local branch of the Samaritans and if they knew its telephone number. There were no sex differences in knowledge of the Samaritans but a non-linear effect by age was seen. Those in their mid- to late-60s knew of the Samaritans most (39%) followed by those between the age of 75 and 79 (25%), those 70-74 (19%), and finally the oldest group, aged 80 and above (15%). As suicide rates increase with age, there is a tendency for those with highest rates to know of the Samaritans least. However, Atkinson notes that the high knowledge among the young-old (those 65-69) may forecast higher knowledge in the future among the old so that those who feel suicidal among the aged and advanced aged of the future may know of the service when it is needed. It was also found that the isolated were the least likely to know about the Samaritans (when compared to the less isolated) as were the widowed and divorced. These groups represent high risks for suicide according to the literature (see e.g., Trout, 1980, reference 3-062; Megenhagen et al., 1980, reference 4-064). Only 11% of those who described themselves as "often lonely" knew about the Samaritans, compared to 23% of the "sometimes lonely" and 31% of the "never lonely." With respect to telephone usage in general, it was seen that the isolated also have poorer access to and more difficulty using telephones than do other groups. It was observed that one-third of these elderly total find it difficult to use the telephone and 40% never use it. The problem for the Samaritans, a suicide prevention scheme, and the old, a high risk group for suicide, therefore, is that few of the old and especially those who need it the most know of the existence of the Samaritans and many of the old have difficulty or never use the primary means of contact with the agency (i.e., the telephone).   Atkinson (p. 488) states that "those who are most likely to commit suicide are least likely to know of the Samaritans and marginally less proficient at using telephones."   The implications of this research are that suicide prevention agencies need to make themselves better known to the old and the aged need better access and familiarity with using telephones. As younger cohorts, who have more telephone availability and familiarity, enter old age it might be predicted that at least the skills and knowledge necessary to access such agencies will increase. Awareness of the availability of such services will remain a need.

4-006   Bagley, Christopher, & Jacobson, Solomon. (1976).   Ecological variation of three types of suicide. Psychological Medicine, 6, 423-427.

This study is a follow-up and extension of Bagley et al. (1976, reference 4-007 below). In that earlier study three subtypes of suicide were determined.   These are labeled by Bagley and Solomon as "old and handicapped," "sociopathic," and "depressed." This investigation looked at 191 suicides in Brighton from two different time periods.   In addition to determining if the three subtypes of suicide can be substantiated with these cases, the authors also hypothesize and find that the different types will live in "ecologically contrasted areas."   The three categories of suicides were observed with these data.

4-007   Bagley, Christopher, Jacobson, Solomon, & Rehin, Ann. (1976). Completed suicide: A taxonomic analysis of clinical and social data. Psychological Medicine, 6, 429-438.

The goal of this investigation was to construct a taxonomy of suicide. A "post-mortem enquiry" was conducted by interviewing relatives of 50 consecutive suicides in Brighton during an eight-month period from 1970-71.   A total of 123 items of information about each case was compiled.   Using various multiple regression analyses, three distinct types or categories of suicide were derived. The first type was "characterized by clinical depression and long-standing psychiatric problems in older, middle-class people" (p. 433), the second by "sociopathic traits in younger individuals who have experienced early deprivation" (p. 433), and the third by "older individuals, enduring chronic pain or physical handicap" (p. 433). Further analyses essentially supported these same categories or clusters of items among 141 cases of Brighton suicides occurring during 1970-1972. For the third type the authors suggest that careful prescribing of medications as well as intervention in the loneliness and effects of physical handicap would likely aid

prevention of suicide among such individuals.   Among   the
depressed group   prevention   efforts should focus on recognition
and treatment   of   depression.   The   authors   admit   that   the
taxonomy derived here is tenative and that most likely more than
three types of suicide occur.

4-008   Batchelor, I. R. C., & Napier, Margaret B. (1953, November   28).
Attempted suicide   in   old   age.   British   Medical   Journal, 2,
1186-1190.

From among a   series   of   200   consecutive   cases   of   attempted
suicide admitted   to   an   Edinburgh   general hospital in 1950 to
1952, 40 (20%) were 60 years of age or above.   These   40   cases
form the   sample   for   the   study   (16   males, 24 females).   The
following described what was discovered about the   sample: 65%
had family   histories   of psychological problems;   17% (N=7) had
family members with suicidal behavior (5 suicides,   2   non-fatal
attempts);   one-fourth had "suffered a fall in social status" in
their lives;   two-thirds were diagnosed as mentally ill;   32 (14
males, 18   females) attempted in a depressive state (higher than
that found in studies of younger age groups);   only   10%   (N=4)
suffered from   organic disorders.   Less than one-fourth of these
attempts were impulsive in nature and more than one-fourth "had
been contemplated   for weeks or months."   Suicidal intention was
immediately admitted by 25 of the 40   while   8   more   denied   at
first but   later   admitted   their suicidal intention.   Only 5 of
the sample denied their suicidal intent while 1 claimed amnesia.
The authors suggest that mental illness is more commonly seen in
elderly sucidal acts than in younger age groups but   they   point
out the multiple etiology of suicide acts for the old as well as
other age   groups.   It is maintained that the motivation for the
old is more likely to include feelings of loneliness (present in
23 of the cases) and increasing physical incapacities (seen   in
18 cases)   while less likely including dramatic gestures, escape
from socially   embarrassing   situations   and   involvement   of
intoxication.   Financial anxiety was a factor in only 6 cases in
this sample.   The authors conclude that when depression develops
in a   predisposed   individual   (family   history   of   suicide and
psychopathology, broken home in   childhood,   etc.) with   lowered
resistance due   to   old   age,   health   problems,   interpersonal
losses, etc.,   that   feelings   of   loneliness,   weariness,   and
despair "may   be   set   in   motion   which   tends   to eventuate in
suicide" (p. 1190).   It is suggested that   promotion   of   mental
health in   young   ages as well as employment as long as possible
coupled with   promoting   other   interests,   increased   social
integration, early   treatment   of   mental   health   problems, and
increased and early recognition of the warning signs in the   old
should lead to fewer elderly suicides.

4-009   Bock, E. Wilbur. (1972).   Aging and suicide: The   significance
of   marital,   kinship,   and   alternative   relations.   Family
Coordinator, 21, 71-79.

This article presents an overview of the findings   of   Bock   and

Webber (1972a, 1972b, references 4-010 & 4-011). The author reviews a variety of social relationships which are hypothesized to maintain external restraints against suicidal behavior (i.e., marriage, kinship networks, and work). The impact of physical illness on social relationships is also discussed. The review of these social relationships led to an investigation of how these varying relations are related to suicidal behavior in the elderly. Data from a Pinellas County, FL field survey of randomly sampled persons aged 65 and over were used as a normative group with which elderly suicides were compared. A total of 188 suicides occurred in Pinellas County from 1955 to 1963 among persons 65 and above. These cases were determined from death certificates and funeral directors' files. Significant relationships between certain types of social relationships and suicide were found, however, marriage in and of itself, was not enough to prevent suicide. Organizational memberships and on-going relationships with family and friends were also reported as important in maintaining life. Substitution of other relationships for those lost through death and other reasons may aid in the reduction of suicide potential. Greater prevention seemed to be found with greater numbers of involvements. Recommendations for prevention include continued targeting of the socially isolated, additional focus on the married elderly who have no other social ties, and an emphasis in incorporating formal organizations into the daily life of the elderly. "Social autopsies" are recommended to provide more complete information on the number, types, and strength of formal and informal social ties engaged in by potential and successful suicides.

4-010   Bock, E. Wilbur, & Webber, Irving L. (1972a). Social status and relational systems of elderly suicides: A reexamination of the Henry-Short thesis. Life-Threatening Behavior, 2, 144-159.

This article presents detailed data on the 188 elderly suicides discussed in Bock (1972, reference 4-009) and Bock and Webber (1972b, reference 4-011) and focuses on social class status and the relational system. Social class status was determined by occupations and classified into categories used by the United States Bureau of the Census. Relational system was based on marital status, location of kin in the same county, and membership in formal organizations. The study tests several hypotheses about social integration and suicide that are derived from the work of Henry and Short (1954, Suicide and Homicide, New York: Free Press). Both social class and relation systems seem to affect suicide rates independently and jointly, but the data indicated a stronger effect upon suicide rates for the strength of the relational system than for social status. Lower class elderly males were found to be particularly at high risk for suicide but the social class-relation system effect on suicide was complex. The authors conclude that those who have fewer meaningful relations with others (e.g., those of lower-class levels) are a primary target for prevention programs as should be generally reinforcing and substituting relationships for those that are lost. The need to investigate information about relationships beyond that available on death certificates, and especially less formal support systems, is noted.

In a comment on this article, Short (1972, Life-Threatening Behavior, 2, 160–162) quotes from Henry and Short (1954) that status and relation system strength "were operating in opposite directions" with regard to the aged. The low status of the old ought to produce low suicide rates but the weak social relations predict high rates. Therefore, Bock and Webber's findings are not so divergent from hypotheses made by Henry and Short for the old and Short is not surprised that the relational system seems to have a stronger effect.

4-011   Bock, E. Wilbur, & Webber, Irving L. (1972b). Suicide among the elderly: Isolating widowhood and mitigating alternatives. Journal of Marriage and the Family, 34, 24–31.

This article presents detailed data on the 188 elderly suicides discussed in Bock (1972, reference 4-009) and Bock and Webber (1972a, reference 4-010) and focuses on the comparison of the widowed vs. the married. The main findings were: (1) the widowed, especially widowers, are more likely than the married to commit suicide. While the suicide rates for widows (females; rate=10.98) and wives (rate=8.06) were similar, though in the direction indicated, widowers (males; rate=80.68) were much larger risks than husbands (rate=23.94). As the authors state (p. 26), "judging from the propensity to self-annihilation, widowhood has particularly devastating results for these elderly widowers." (2) The differences between widowers and the other groups are partially due to social isolation. There were no differences between wives and widows for having relatives in the community and belonging to organizations, but widowers were less likely to have both (but especially the latter) than were wives, widows, or husbands. Widows, though they also had lost a spouse, were more likely to be involved in alternative relations and to be members in organizations. (3) Strong relational systems can have a stronger effect than marital status alone with respect to suicide rates. That is, widows and widowers with strong or medium relational systems have lower suicide rates than wives or husbands with weak relational systems. (4) Widows may find alternative relations to lessen suicide likelihood, but widowers have many fewer possibilities. Thus, while alternatives to the marriage relation may counter suicide, widowers are more limited in the degree to which the loss can be so mitigated. The authors conclude that prevention programs need to pay special attention to widowers.

4-012   Burston, G. R. (1969). Self-poisoning in elderly patients. Gerontologia Clinica, 11, 279–289.

This article describes data for the 33 elderly patients (from among 505 total patients of all ages) treated for self-poisoning

(deliberate or accidental consumption) at a North-East England
infirmary from October 1966 to March 1968. The subjects
consisted of 8 males (Mean age=76.9; range=70-88) and 25
females (Mean age=68.2; range=60-81). Compared to the patients
younger than 60 for females and less than 65 for males, these 33
elderly patients (1) had made more serious acts, as seen by much
higher levels of unconsciousness when admitted (34% were
classified as severely self-poisoned compared to only 18% of the
younger patients). (2) The elderly patients used different
methods of self-poisoning, preferring barbiturates and coal gas
while the young employed salicylates and "other drugs" most
often. Among the elderly, 23% used more than one type of drug
in their self-poisoning. (3) The elderly patients stayed on the
unit an average of 7 days compared to only 3 for the young, and
(4) psychiatric management of the old patients following the
initial treatment and discharge were very similar to the young
self-poisoners.

The immediate precipitating cause for the self-poisoning act was
most often depression (45%), followed by personal (or others')
physical health problems (25%), loneliness (20%), and accidental
self-poisonings or "gestures" (10%). A brief case example for
each of the major causes is included. A mail follow-up survey
of the patients' general practitioners (response rate=94%)
indicated that 68% were still alive, and among those who had
died, none had died from suicide or made other attempts prior to
their death (from 2 weeks to 9 months after the original
self-poisoning). Apparently no further attempts at the
follow-up had occurred among the living patients either. The
author also notes that only 13% of these elderly patients had
indicated their intention to kill themselves to relatives prior
to their self-poisoning. Vague warning signs were often
recognized by relatives after the attempt however. Many had
"bought" the myth that those who talk about death (and suicide)
will not kill themselves. It is noted that many self-poisoning
elderly, though representing a small proportion of all cases,
have correctable physical illness that should be treated while
hospitalized. The author concludes with the statement that
"Some of these episodes appear to be an attempt to forstall an
unpleasant impending death in those elderly patients with
chronic ill health" (p. 288).

4-013   Brown, James H., Henteleff, Paul, Barakat, Samia, & Rowe, Cheryl
        J. (1986). Is it normal for terminally ill patients to desire
        death? American Journal of Psychiatry, 143, 208-211.

This investigation was undertaken in an attempt to better
understand whether "people faced with serious life problems,
especially people with painful, disfiguring, or disabling
terminal illness" (p. 208) seriously consider suicide or wish to
die. The literature on the topic is scarce with mixed results.
A sample of 331 consecutive patients was selected for possible
participation in the study from among those patients of a
hospice-principled general hospital in Canada. Those with

terminal illness, pain, severe disfigurement, and/or severe disability, and awareness of the nature of their illness and its prognosis were included in the 331 while those excluded had organic mental impairment, an inability to communicate, an inability to give informed consent, or were too sick. As a result of the exclusion criteria, only 50 of the 331 patients were interviewed and six more were eliminated for various reasons. This left 44 patients, 22 males and 22 females, who were interviewed and completed the short form of the Beck Depression Inventory. Mean age was 63 years with a range from 29 to 82 years. Most of the patients had some form of carcinoma. Results showed that 34 of the 44 had never thought of suicide or wished to die early and none asked for mercy killing. One patient was currently expressing suicidal ideation, two had been formerly but not presently suicidal, while seven desired currently or in the past for death but not for suicide. All of those who desired death suffered from severe depression. From among all 44 patients, 11 were severely depressed, including the 10 cited above. "The striking feature of these results is that all of the patients who had either desired premature death or contemplated suicide were judged to be suffering from clinical depressive illness" (p. 210). The 25% proportion of severely depressed among these 44 patients is higher than in the general population but their psychological and physical circumstances make these levels understandable. "It would appear [from these findings] that patients with terminal illness who are not mentally ill are no more likely than the general population to wish for premature death" (p. 210). The results of this investigation have methodological difficulties and the generalization of these findings should be carefully considered, but the results have implications for the recent controversy over "rational suicide," especially among terminally ill individuals. Further research into this topic is warranted.

4-014 Cahn, L. A. (1966). Suicide and attempted suicide in old age. Proceedings: Seventh International Congress of Gerontology (pp. 43-45). Vienna: Wiener Medizinischen Akademie.

Cahn describes old age as a time of crisis, "a period wherein man must fight to maintain himself despite decreased mental, physical and material reserves" (p. 43). Suicide then is a possible response to these crises. Cahn also states that "Suicide can therefore not be seen apart from the reaction it evokes in others" (p. 44). The study related in this paper involved 107 persons over age 65 who were admitted to a psychiatric department for attempted suicide. There were twice as many men as women in the group and social factors were important motivations for the attempt for 40% of the men. The lonely old person and the widower are singled out as very high risks for suicidal behavior. Of the 107 cases, 75% appeared to result from a reaction to a trauma or stress while in the other 25% psychological disorders were important. Paranoid psychosis was observed in over half of the cases. Cahn suggests therefore, that "It is fear that has brought these people to suicide. They fear to be killed by others. Those others will let them starve, will rob them of everything" (p. 45). The loneliness and insecurity then are seen as major factors in these attempts. It is noted that the later period of life is different than younger periods and the events taking place there must be understood with respect to their meaning at that time.

4-015 Cameron, Paul. (1972).   Suicide   and   the   generation   gap. Life-Threatening Behavior, 2, 194-208.

This study looked at the beliefs about those of various ages with regard to suicidal behavior among young adults (18-25 years), middle-aged (40-55), and old (65-79) adults. A sample of 317 individuals from the city of Detroit of the above ages and of each sex was recruited by visits to their homes and telephone calls. All of the age groups believed that the old (1) have the greatest wish to die, (2) knew the least about suicide, (3) make the fewest attempted suicides, (4) are least often successful in their attempts, and (5) are least condemned for committing suicide. The subjects also responded to self-appraisals and there were no differences among the age groups with respect to the consideration of suicide or suicide attempts. The beliefs of these groups are clearly not consistent with the data that exist on suicide completions (point 4 above). As the author states, "All generations agreed that suicide among young adults is the most condemned, while among the old it is the easiest excused" (p. 205).

4-016 Chia, Boon H. (1979). Suicide of the elderly in Singapore. Annals of the Academy of Medicine of Singapore, 8, 290-297.

Trends and characteristics of suicides in Singapore age 60 and above are presented for 1957-1977 with detailed data from coroner's case files for 1969-1977 (539 cases). Great fluctuation but high rates was noted over the period of study for both sexes. Rates for elderly males were higher than for females (1974-1977 rates were 64.1 and 31.9, respectively). No increase in rates was observed for either sex and a downward trend was seen for elderly males (the high risk for males above age 60 continues in 1980 data as well, see Ee Heok Kua & Wing Foo Tsoi, Suicide in the island of Singapore, Acta Psychiatrica Scandinavica, 1985, 71, 227-229). Unlike U.S. suicide, rates peak in old age for both sexes in Singapore. Overrepresentation among the suicidal elderly (compared to characteristics of the aged Singapore population as a whole) were found for the nonmarried population (divorced, widowed, separated included), Chinese (compared to Indian and Malay populations), the unemployed, and the foreign-born. The commonest method for all age groups was jumping from high-rise flats but the most common for elderly males was hanging while elderly females employed drowning and poisoning more often than males. Among all age groups, the elderly of both sexes had made the fewest previous attempts so that the fatal attempt was usually the first and last. The aged also least often wrote suicide notes. The notes of the old were brief, less often expressed affect (either positive or negative), and tended to contain neutral instructions. Notes by those under 24 "were reproachful and filled with self-criticism, self-hate, and self-pity" (p. 293). The author also looked more closely at the 57 cases (39 males, 18 females) of suicides occurring in 1974 who were over 60 years of age. These individuals (a) most often lived in the lower social strata; (b) the majority were mentally ill; (c) more males (80%) than females (33%) were physically ill; (d) almost none (only 1 male and 1 female) had received psychiatric care while 80% of the males and 44% of the females had received medical care prior to their suicide; (e) about one-third of male and female elderly had economic problems that were associated with their suicides and more female than male suicides were associated with interpersonal conflicts. Only 5% of these elderly suicides of both sexes had terminal cancer.

This study also assessed the reactions of the relatives ("survivors") of the 1974 aged suicides. It was observed that (a) about one-third (35%) of the survivors were surprised at the news of the suicide despite frequent clues to suicide ideation, (b) 31% felt the mode of death was shameful, (c) many (46%) had depressive feelings and (d) shame (33%), (e) while 15% worried about neighbors' gossip. "Surprisingly, feelings of guilt, seemed to be demonstrated only among the relatives of female suicides (22%)" (p. 296). Chia suggested that "relatives, especially the sons and daughters, were afraid that others would feel that they had not done their duty toward their old folk, or that they had been unfilial" (p. 297).

4-017   Chynoweth, Ray. (1981). Suicide in the elderly. Crisis: International Journal of Suicide- and Crisis-Studies, 2, 106-116.

This article presents official data on elderly suicide for Australia from 1961-1974 and detailed data for Brisbane, Queensland during 1973-1974. As seen in the U.S.A., males 65 and above had the highest rates of any male age grouping. For females, on the other hand, rates peak between 35 and 64 and are much less for those over 65. Elderly male rates are approximately three times those of elderly females. While a general trend toward decreased rates of suicide is seen for both sexes above 65, there has been much less change for males over the period of study.

Among the 135 suicides in Brisbane from 1973-1974, 24 (13.3%) were above age 60 and are reported in detail. Significant differences between the younger and old suicides include: (1) a higher proportion of widowed among the old. (2) Only two factors related to depressive symptomatology, namely, (a) increased feelings of guilt among elderly females, and (b) increased hypochondriacal ideas among elderly males. (3) No differences among age groups were found in the proportions having a past history of mental illness, previous suicide attempts, family history of psychiatric disorders, and history of alcohol and/or drug dependence problems (33%, 29%, 17%, 13%, respectively among the over 60 suicides). (4) Physical disease was more often seen among the old (35% of 39 and below suicides, 59% of 40–59, 71% of 60+) and more often contributed to the suicide (25%, 27%, 54% among the age groups, respectively). By sex, active and contributing illness was present in 64% of the male and 46% of the female elderly suicides. (5) The use of drugs and alcohol were important problems for the young but not for the old, although the old were more likely to be receiving prescribed drugs. Prescribed drugs were more often used among elderly female suicides than the other groups. (6) The old had seen a physician recently more often than had the young. A total of 71% of the elderly suicides had seen a physician within 4 weeks of their death and 17% had done so within one week. (7) The old (38%) were more likely to be alone at the time of the suicide, but about two-thirds of the elderly suicides were <u>not</u> living alone.

While males presented to physicians with physical symptoms most frequently, females presented with anxiety. The author concludes that to lower elderly suicides, that elderly male patients with physical disorders need to be followed up more frequently and assessment of depression made so that medication can be provided. For aged females the need to recognize depression is also noted as is the need for social support.

4-018 Ciompi, Luc. (1976). Late suicide in former mental patients. <u>Psychiatria Clinica</u>, <u>9</u>, 59–63. (Abstracts found in: <u>Community Mental Health Review</u>, 1977, <u>2</u>(3), No. 200, p. 14; and <u>Psychological Abstracts</u>, 1977, <u>58</u>, No. 7622, p. 811)

This study presents the results of long-term follow-up in their old age of 1,891 former Swiss mental patients. The 1891 individuals represent those who had died by the follow-up. Of these deaths, 107 (5.6%) were deaths by suicide. The rates of suicide among all the diagnostic groups were higher than for the Swiss general population of the same age. The author summarizes by stating that "former mental patients of all kinds constitute a specific high-risk group for suicide in old age."

4-019 Darbonne, A. R. (1969). Suicide and age: A suicide note analysis. <u>Journal of Consulting and Clinical Psychology</u>, <u>33</u>, 46–50.

Darbonne analyzed 259 notes written by 156 individuals for five general categories of content (addressee, reasons stated, affect indicated, specific content, general focus of note). Four age categories are considered and sample suicide notes for each age group are included. The number of notes in each age category and by sex is omitted. The notes represent all such notes written during a 3-year period in 34 moderately advantaged Los Angeles communities (representing "average" LA communities). Of of various ages, notes of young adults (20–39) more often than older suicide notes indicated feelings of rejection and heterosexual relationship problems. There was a general absence of illness and pain as reasons and less frequent asking for forgiveness. The affect that was present was one of love and affection for others with internalized blame, guilt, and self-depreciation. The notes of 40–49 year olds were "a communication of the vanquished. They seemed unequal to the demands of life and were tired or bored and wanted a way out. They entered the period of the change of life already stating that they had reached the end and couldn't go on" (p. 49). The 50–59 year olds were least likely of all age groups to indicate a reason for their suicide (while those over 60 were most likely). Instead, their notes gave instructions and unemotional information and messages. Much less affect was noted in the notes of this older middle age group. Darbonne conjectured that perhaps these individuals had "arrived at the conclusion that others would not care or understand their feelings," (p. 49) or possibly their actions resulted from rational, well-conceived decisions that death was the correct choice. Those note writers 60 and above more often than any other age group gave answers to the question "why?". Reasons most often cited included illness, pain, physical disability, loneliness and isolation. Expressions of sorrow and forgiveness were frequently present but there was an absence of feelings of self-depreciation and guilt. Interestingly, this group indicated no more often than other groups that they were tired of life and nearly absent from all age groups were financial motivations or confusion/psychotic thoughts. Only about 14–25% of suicides leave notes and it is possible that there are group differences in this proportion. Therefore, the representativeness of note writers to all suicides of the above ages is not known and should be kept in mind.

4-020   De Catanzaro, Denys. (1984). Suicidal ideation and the residual capacity to promote inclusive fitness: A survey. Suicide and Life-Threatening Behavior, 14, 74–87.

This article details a study conducted to test a biosocial theory of suicide put forth by the author (more detailed presentation of the theory may be found in: Human suicide: A biological perspective. Behavioral and Brain Sciences, 1980, 3, 264–290, and Suicide and Self-Damaging Behavior: A Sociobiological Perspective, 1981, New York: Academic Press). A major argument of the theory is that "suicide generally occurs among individuals whose residual capacity to promote their inclusive fitness is diminished. . . . inclusive fitness encompasses his own welfare and reproductive potential and those of his kin" (p. 76). For groups like the elderly which include individuals who perceive their coming (remaining) years to be ones in which their ability to contribute is diminished, suicide should therefore be high.

The study was a survey of two populations. Three regions of

Ontario, Canada were chosen and 1000 questionnaires sent to each region to individuals selected from local telephone directories. Of the 3000 questionnaires sent out, 717 were returned (24%) and 711 were usable. Respondents ranged in age from 18-88 with a mean age of 40.72 years. Of this sample, 4.36% had attempted suicide at some time in their lives. A second sample was chosen from among undergraduates at McMaster University. Class sections were selected from among those listed in the registration materials and faculty of 16 of 20 sections chosen allowed distribution and completion of the survey questionnaire to their classes. A total of 825 students (mean age=21.22) participated with 821 usable questionnaires. Only 2.44% of these students had previously attempted suicide.

The survey consisted of 57 questions asking basic personal and relationship information as well as questions on suicidal ideation and behavior, and attitudes about the value of life. Results were overall very similar for both samples and generally supported the theory advanced. The young reported more suicidal ideation than did the old. Multiple regression analyses were performed for several groupings including 51-88 years (N=193). Among this age group, suicidal ideation was best predicted by the four variables (questions/ratings) regarding "My family would be better off without me," "current health," "past contribution to society," and "expectation of future sexual relationship" (among males). De Catanzaro suggests that it is not just reproductive ability that must be considered in inclusive fitness. It is possible, though not necessarily sufficient, to gain (lessen suicidal ideation) through contributions to others and the community.

4-021   De Grove, William. (1979). A three-factor path model of Florida suicide rates. Social Science and Medicine, 13A, 183-185.

This study explores the relevance of Bagley and Jacobson's (1976, reference 4-006) taxonomy of suicide which included (1) old and handicapped, (2) sociopathic, and (3) depressed, as well as Durkheim's concepts of egoism and anomie. De Grove identified three factors in an earlier cross-sectional study (An assessment of community suicide risk, Suicide and Life-Threatening Behavior, 1977, 7, 100-107) of white suicide rates in 24 Florida counties, which he interpreted as representative of isolation, anomie, and psychopathology. He felt these were parallel to Bagley and Jacobson's types, with "isolation" the same as "old and handicapped." The relationship of age to these three factors is discussed and it is concluded that the relative effects of age upon isolation, anomie, and psychopathology must be considered in analysis. Controlling for age of the subject, path analysis was used to test De Grove's three factor model. The author concludes the taxonomy (isolation, anomie, psychopathology) proposed by Bagley and Jacobson was supported by the suicide rates in Florida. He summed the results of the path analyses as: "In Florida, the age structure of the population is the dominant factor in area

suicide rates; however, after age is taken into consideration
anomie, isolation, and psychopathology appear in that order as
causal factors" (p. 185). Controlled study of individual
suicides was recommended.

4-022 Dorpat, Theodore L., Anderson, William F., & Ripley, Herbert
S. (1968). The relationship of physical illness to suicide. In
H. L. P. Resnik (Ed.), Suicidal behaviors: Diagnosis and
management (pp. 209-219). Boston: Little, Brown.

This study was conducted to determine the role physical illness
plays in attempted and completed suicide. The samples of
completed and attempted suicides were taken from those in King
County, Washington. A total of 114 suicides occurred during a
one year period in the county and 80 had sufficient information
regarding illness to be included in the study. Data were
gathered from interviews with friends and relatives, physicians,
and hospital and police records. The attempted sample was 60
consecutive cases at the county hospital that the law required
all attempted suicides to be admitted to for psychiatric
service. Psychiatric interviews as well as information from
family and friends were employed for the attempters. It was
determined if physical illness contributed to the suicide or
attempt by its effect on the individual. Among the 80 completed
suicides, 56 (70%) had active illness(es) at the time of their
suicide and in 41 of those 56 the illness(es) was felt to have
contributed to the suicide. For the 60 attempted suicides,
medical histories for 58 were available and among these 58, 20
(34.5%) had active physical illness(es) at the time of their
attempt, with 18 (31%) of the illnesses considered a
contributing factor. When broken down by age, physical illness
was found to be the most common precipitating factor for those
60 years of age and older and the old had active physical illess
significantly more often than the other age groups among the
completed suicides. For those 60 and above 84.8% had active
illness, compared to 68.8% for those aged 40-59, and 40% for
those under 40. No statistically significant age difference was
found for physical illness among the attempters. For the sample
as a whole, males who committed suicide had significantly
greater illness than did females but there were no sex
differences among attempters. Several extremely brief case
examples are presented to illustrate various motivations to
suicide or attempted suicide. Some of the examples are for
elderly individuals. For the old, the authors conclude that
physical illness may threaten employment and it produces greater
isolation and loneliness. With respect to the entire sample,
"For many, illness meant the approach of death, which they
feared. Rather than wait and passively experience death they
sought to master their fear of death by actively bringing about
their own demise" (p. 219).

4-023 Farberow, Norman L., & Moriwaki, Sharon Y. (1975).
Self-destructive crises in the older person. Geontologist, 15,
333-337. (Reprinted in Garry L. Landreth & Robert C. Berg

(Eds.) (1980), Counseling the elderly: For professional helpers
who   work   with   the   aged   (pp. 342–349).   Springfield,   IL:
Thomas.)

This report presents data on elderly suicides in Veterans
Administration populations, general medical and surgical
patients [GM&S], and older neuropsychiatric hospital patients
[NP]. In addition, data on older adults who call suicide
prevention centers are presented, specifically for the Los
Angeles center.   The authors found that suicides in NP were
younger (mean age=39.1) than in GM&S settings (mean=52.3).   In
addition, 18% of the GM&S hospital suicides during the period
1970–1972 were 60 or older while 7% of the NP patient suicides
were 60 or more (the aged represented 26% and 23% of the patient
populations in general, respectively).   It is suggested that NP
patients have been hospitalized for more of their lives and have
adapted to institutions.   Elderly suicides in both settings were
characterized by   multiple   problems.   Apparently   the
"accumulation of losses becomes so distressing that they prefer
to end their lives" (p. 334). The methods employed to commit
suicide reflect the availability of methods in the two settings.
Since NP settings usually have screens and grilles on the
windows patients most often employ objects with which they can
hang themselves.   Most GM&S hospitals do not have such window
hardware and jumping was the most common method.   The suicides
in both settings share the use of highly lethal methods as well
as their apparent lack of warning signs or clues to their intent
to kill themselves.

The authors next present information on callers to the Los
Angeles Suicide Prevention Center for 1973–1974 who were 60 and
above. From the first 8000 calls received, the old represented
only about 300 or 2.6%, indicating the underrepresentativeness
of older individuals among the callers.   While the old and those
of younger ages called the center in such proportions that
two–thirds of the callers were female and one–third males, the
authors note that this is significant for the old.   Because
women are overrepresented in the old population while there are
nearly equal proportions of the sexes in the general population,
the one–third men among the old who called the center indicates
that higher proportions of men are calling among the old than
the young. "Men are now reaching out and asking for help more
frequently than when young.   It is possible the culture makes
fewer demands . . . of the elderly person" (p. 335) is one
possible explanation.   The widowed and especially widowers were
found to be overrepresented among the callers over 60 who called
during the first 4 months of 1974 when compared to the
proportions in the aged population as a whole. "Those who call
have fewer social resources and support" (p. 335).   Men
indicated that they were considering more lethal methods than
did women callers. The reasons for calling for men were: 26%
depression, 18% physical illness, 18% grief and loneliness over
the loss of a loved one. For women the proportions were 29%,
22%, and 29%, respectively.   These people called the suicide

prevention center as a result of a crisis that was taking place for the individual who already had high levels of distress. Brief clinical vignettes that illustrate typical cases in GM&S, NP, and suicide prevention center settings are presented. The authors conclude by suggesting that many elderly may not call suicide prevention centers because of the name. That is, they may be lonely, unhappy, etc., but not necessarily suicidal and therefore the service seems inappropriate. It is also possible, as Atkinson (1971, reference 4-005) observed in Britain, that the old are not aware of the existence of the centers or are less able to use or access telephones to make the contact. To improve the likelihood that the old will call crisis services, the authors suggest that a telephone specifically targeted and identified as for the aged be developed. The center should be staffed by those trained to understand the problems of the aged and the appropriate agencies for intervention. Some of these individuals may be themselves elderly. Finally, such a center, to be maximally effective and likely to produce preventive efforts, should include an outreach program.

4-024   Farberow, Norman L., & Shneidman, Edwin S. (1970). Suicide and age. In Edwin S. Shneidman, Norman L. Farberow, & Robert E. Litman (Eds.), The psychology of suicide (pp. 164-174). New York: Science House. (Reprinted from Edwin S. Shneidman & Norman L. Farberow (Eds.). (1957), Clues to suicide (pp. 41-49). New York: McGraw-Hill.)

The authors address the question of differing dynamics in varying age groups of suicidal persons. A sample of 619 suicide notes obtained from the Los Angeles County, CA Coroner's office was examined. The suicide notes were collected from 1944 to 1953 and all writers were native-born Caucasians. Males (N=489) ranged in age from 20-96 and females (N=130) from 20-78. Karl Menninger's theory of suicide, which broadly characterizes psychodynamic motivations underlying suicide into three categories (i.e., the wish to kill, the wish to be killed, the wish to die), was selected for analysis of the suicide notes. The notes were grouped according to the age of the writer (20-39=young, 40-49=middle-aged, 60-96=old) and Menninger's three groups or an unclassified grouping if the note contained insufficient information to determine suicidal category. Representative notes from the various age and suicidal classifications are presented. The factor of the wish to die increased with age, particularly for males. Anger (the wish to kill or be killed), on the other hand, decreased dramatically as the men aged. Women tended to express about the same amount of anger throughout the life span, but the older women's suicide notes expressed less guilt and self-blame and more despair and discouragement than among younger women. The authors caution the reader about the conclusions as 23% of the male notes and 19% of the female notes were unclassifiable. An additional caution is made that the sample may not be representative of all suicides because it represents only note writers (who comprise only about 15% of the suicides in Los Angeles). Recommendations

for therapeutic treatment of varying age groups are made. For
the old it is suggested that relief of physical pain and
supportive treatment aimed at relieving depressive symptoms may
be helpful.

4-025   Ford, Amasa B., Rushforth, Norman B., Rushforth, Nancy, Hirsch,
Charles S., & Adelson, Lester. (1979). Violent death in a
metropolitan county: II. Changing patterns in suicides
(1959-1974). American Journal of Public Health, 69, 459-464.

A study of 3264 suicides over a 17-year period (1958-1974) in
Cuyahoga County, OH (which includes Cleveland) is detailed by
age, sex, and race. As found for the nation as a whole, suicide
rates increased for the young and declined for the old (for both
sexes), but rates by age remained highest among the elderly and
especially elderly white males. Race and sex differences
overall and by age also mirrored those for the nation as a whole
as did the increasing use of firearms by all age-sex-race
groups. Rates were higher in the city areas than in the
suburbs. Of the suicides from 1969-1974, 20.2% (203/1006) of
those who were "dead on arrival" had blood alcohol levels of
0.1% or greater, and the percentage increased from the earliest
years of the study period. The authors suggest the following
changes which may have reduced stress (and suicide) during the
time period of study for the old: "increased access to
hospitals for older persons since 1965 Medicare legislation, the
development of somewhat improved social services for the aged,
and the enlargement of social and political action associations
among the older persons themselves" (p. 463).

4-026   Gardner, Elmer A., Bahn, Anita K., & Mack, Marjorie. (1964).
Suicide and psychiatric care in the aging. Archives of General
Psychiatry, 10, 547-553.

This study was conducted in an attempt to assist psychiatric
residents in predicting suicidal behavior from the patient's
psychiatric diagnosis, previous suicide attempts, and
sociological data collected through a New York psychiatric
register of Monroe County, NY during 1960-1962. Those over 55
years of age represented 20 of the 54 cases (case=individual
with known psychiatric contact). Older suicides were more
likely to have been seen as inpatients while the younger were
more often treated as outpatients. The authors report that both
successful and attempted suicides often seek help before their
suicidal act. Persons diagnosed with affective psychoses had
the highest suicide rate, second highest were neurotic or
personality disorders, with patients with chronic brain
syndromes exhibiting the lowest suicide rates. Two psychiatric
populations were singled out as especially high-risk groups:
alcoholics and younger, primarily male, patients diagnosed as
paranoid schizoprhenics. It was noted that the rates after age
55 were twice as high as under 55 for affective psychoses and
neurotic or personality disorders. The authors suggest that
this indicates that depression is common among the old and the

symptomatology often missed. Sociologically, five factors
emerged for the older compared to younger suicides: (1) older
adult (primarily male) living in lower SES area, (2) low-status
occupation, downward job mobility, lack of employment, (3)
single, separated, divorced, widowed, living alone (social
isolation), (4) physical illness, and (5) no regular contact
with friends or relatives. The authors recommend that
clinicians pay more attention to elderly depression (which may
be masked by denial, organic deterioration, or disengagement),
potential for loss of control over their lives, and
environmental and sociocultural factors (e.g., isolation,
illness, etc.) in their patients' history.

4-027   Gerifacts: Suicide patterns in the elderly. (1967, December).
        Geriatrics, 22, 68.

This brief statistical perspective presents official suicide
data for the year 1964. Although elderly suicide declined since
1950 (to 1964), suicide rates among persons aged 44-64 remain
high enough to make suicide one of the ten leading causes of
death in this age group. Suicide rates for white males over 60
remain high (over 40 per 100,000 population and 65.1 for white
males over age 85). White and nonwhite females reach a suicidal
peak between ages 45 and 64 and then the suicide rate steadily
declines. Nonwhite males exhibit an irregular pattern that
increases slightly from 45 to 75 and then drops sharply (compare
this to patterns noted for nonwhites in later data years in
McIntosh, 1984, reference 4-059). Marital status also affects
suicide rates, with elderly married individuals having the
lowest overall rate, but showing a marked rise after age 60.
Suicide rates may, in truth, be twice the reported figures due
to the reluctance to admit the suicidal intent of friends and
neighbors. Ambiguous circumstances surrounding some deaths also
may cause underreporting.

4-028   Gibbs, Jack P., & Martin, Walter T. (1964). Status integration
        and suicide: A sociological study. Eugene: University of
        Oregon Books.

A sociological theory that attempts to predict differences (and
expected rank orders) between suicide rates of groups is
proposed and tested. The theory is an attempt to more clearly
define and allow measurement of Durkheim's (1897/1951, reference
3-014) concept of "social integration" and its effect on
suicide. The major theorem of Gibbs and Martin's theory is "The
suicide rate of a population varies inversely with the degree of
status integration in that population" (p. 27). The authors
systematically test their theory among various race, age, sex,
and marital status categories using U.S. and European suicide
data and measures of status integration. Chapter 6 (pp. 67-77)
is the main consideration of age and suicide. Using measures of
occupation as the indicator of status integration, the major
theorem can be restated such that an inverse relationship should
be found between suicide rates by age and integration of

occupation by age. Therefore, the old, who are typically not employed, have low occupational integration and should exhibit high levels of suicide compared to age groups with higher occupational integration. Data for white males in particular were especially supportive of the theory, but in general the theory predicted well the rank order of suicide rates among age-sex-race groupings.

4-029   Goldney, Robert D., & Katsikitis, Mary. (1983). Cohort analysis of suicide rates in Australia. Archives of General Psychiatry, 40, 71-74.

Cohort analyses (following the suicide rates of birth cohorts as they age) were conducted for official Australian suicide data from 1951 to 1979. By following 5-year birth cohorts beginning with those 15-19 from 1951-1955 (and looking at mean rates for subsequent 5-year intervals), six time periods were derived from the 1951-1979 data for the above cohort. Subsequent 5-year data representing birth cohorts were followed through the period as well. The study revealed an increase in suicide rates for each cohort as it aged. In addition, for the 14-19 and 20-24 aged periods of each cohort, successive cohorts were found to have higher rates than their predecessors at these ages. These findings in general agree with those of data for the U.S. (Murphy & Wetzel, 1980, reference 4-069) and Alberta, Canada (Solomon & Hellon, 1980, reference 4-094). Among older cohorts, for which more complete data are currently available into old age, Goldney and Katsikitis note the "leveling off and slight reduction of suicide rates for the older age cohorts" (p. 74) occurring in the 1960s and 1970s. They suggest these reductions may have been due to the lessened availability of methods of suicide in Australia, particularly the amount of barbiturates prescribed, as a result of legislation in 1967. Methodological differences in the data considered in these cohort analyses studies are presented while cautions and the need for further study regarding current and future data are also noted.

4-030   Gove, Walter R., & Hughes, Michael. (1980). Reexamining the ecological fallacy: A study in which aggregate data are critical in investigating the pathological effects of living alone. Social Forces, 58, 1157-1177.

Methodological issues and controversy surrounding the "ecological fallacy" (i.e., the use of aggregate data to infer about individual cases) are discussed. The argument is made that in the case of the effects of living alone on suicide the only appropriate data with which to make inferences about individuals are aggregate in nature. It is hypothesized that living alone plays an important role in suicide death (and alcoholism). The authors suggest that "the same personality and behavioral problems that lead them to live alone" lead also to suicide (and alcoholism). The average suicide rate for the three-year period 1969-1971 was employed as the dependent or "predicted" variable. Among the independent and control variables was percent living alone. When looking at the independent (i.e., unique) variance contributed by each variable, age, percent of the population of low education, percent of the population with low income, percent of the population that is nonwhite, and population size were unrelated to the suicide rate. Although not strongly, persons per square mile significantly contributed but in a direction opposite to expectations (i.e., a negative relationship). It was suggested that urbanization is now and has been for some time the norm in most Western societies, and the peoples of these cultures have adapted to it and the stress it involves. Percent living alone was the most powerful suicide rate predictor variable, accounting for over one-third of the total explained variance. The percent of the population unemployed was also a significant predictor but was much weaker than percent living alone. The authors argue that their data support a causal link between living alone and suicide and suggest that the effects are due to social isolation. Society is experiencing increasing numbers of individuals living alone, particularly among the elderly population. This group appears to be at high risk for a number of social pathologies, among them suicide.

In a comment on Gove and Hughes' article, Warren Handel (1981, The danger of committing the ecological fallacy persists: Comment on Gove and Hughes, Social Forces, 60, 584–588) points out that aggregate data consistently show correlations between the percentage of persons living alone in a community and suicide and/or alcoholism rates. Causal attributions are often inferred. However, the alternative explanation that suicide may be caused by living in a social environment with other persons who live alone is an equally possible etiological factor, as aggregate data prohibit distinguishing between the two possibilities. Handel criticizes Gove and Hughes for rejecting the latter hypothesis, and dismisses their conclusions as methodologically invalid. Research related to the extent to which behaviors around an individual determine his/her behavior is discussed, and the notion of dismissing a phenomena one is unable to discover in the literature derided.

4-031   Hafner, H., & Schmidtke, A. (1985). Do cohort effects influence suicide rates? [Letter to the Editor]. Archives of General Psychiatry, 42, 926–927.

In response to cohort analysis studies published in this journal (Goldney & Katsikitis, 1983, reference 4-029; Murphy & Wetzel, 1980, reference 4-069; Solomon & Hellon, 1980, reference 4-094), the present authors briefly discuss birth cohort suicide data for the Federal Republic of Germany (FRG) as well as Switzerland and Sweden. The data were tested for evidence consistent with the other studies in which a "monotonically increasing trend of the suicide rates for successive birth cohorts" (p. 926) was observed. The results suggest increasing suicide rates for FRG males of most age groups but less of an

effect for women. <u>No</u> such increase was found for either sex in
Sweden although it was apparent in both sexes for Switzerland.
Further investigation is suggested as to the birth cohort effect
regarding suicide rates by age.

4-032   Hellon, Charles P., & Solomon, Mark I. (1980). Suicide and age
in Alberta, Canada, 1951 to 1977:   The changing profile.
<u>Archives of General Psychiatry</u>, <u>37</u>, 504–510.

As in the U.S., Alberta's suicide rates by age in 1951 exhibited
increases with age and peaks in old age for males, with middle
age peaks followed by declines in old age for females. Over
time, however, there has been little change in the rates for
those over 30 years of age and even declines for those over 60,
while the rates and proportions among total suicides for those
14–29 have increased dramatically. These rates have produced a
profile that by the end of the period of study was better
characterized for both sexes as a peak in young adulthood
followed by declines in rates with increasing age and a second
peak comparable to that in young adulthood in later life. The
authors note the need to understand the reasons for these
changes.

4-033   Holinger, Paul C., & Offer, Daniel. (1982).   Prediction of
adolescent suicide: A population model. <u>American Journal of
Psychiatry</u>, <u>139</u>, 302–307.

This article indeed predominantly presents data regarding
adolescent   suicide   increases.   The authors focus only on
population changes in regard to adolescent suicides (14–19 years
of age). As a comparison group, the 64–69 year old suicide
rates   are also included because they are declining.   A
significant positive relation was found between adolescent
suicide rates and adolescent population percent such that the
fewer adolescents, the fewer adolescent suicides.   For older
adults, on the other hand, although a "trend" toward an inverse
relation was seen, no significant increase or decrease in
suicide was associated with the rise in the percent of the
population comprised by those 64–69. Therefore, the increased
proportion of old in the population in the future would not
necessarily suggest increases (or decreases) in the rate of
elderly suicide.   The tendency for an inverse relation between
population and suicide for the old, however, was addressed by
the authors.   They stated that "the greater number of older
people would not lead to increased competitiveness and failure,
as with the adolescents, but rather to greater attention and
benefits" (p. 306).   The government may pay more economic
attention to the old and the loneliness the suicidal feel may
also decrease with increasing numbers of the old.

4-034   Jarvis, George K., & Boldt, Menno. (1980). Suicide in the later
years. <u>Essence</u>, <u>4</u>, 144–158.

Jarvis and Boldt compare older (N=154, over 60) versus middle

aged (N=611, 30–59) and young suicides (N=366, 14–29) occurring
in Alberta, Canada from 1968 to 1973.   Coroner's files (which
included medical reports, police investigations and interviews
with significant others of the suicide) of officially recorded
suicide deaths were the data source. The elderly suicides were
more likely than young and middle aged suicides to have been
under a physician's treatment at the time of the death, to have
a chronic physical condition,   to   have   physical   illness
attributed as a contributing factor by survivors, to have lived
alone (if they were a male),   and   to have used more lethal
methods to kill themselves.   The old suicides, however, were
less likely to have been drinking or have drugs in their blood
at the time of their death or to have a history of alcoholism or
drug addiction, and to have communicated their intention to
commit suicide or leave a suicide note. "Our findings strongly
suggest that our approach to prevention of suicide among the
elderly must involve a study of the place occupied in the social
system by the older person, as well as greater cognizance of his
or her special needs" (p. 157).

4-035   Jedlicka, Davor. (1978, August).   Suicide and adaptation to
        aging in more developed countries. Paper presented for the 11th
        International Congress of Gerontology, Tokyo, Japan. (Abstract
        appears in Ageing International, the information bulletin of the
        International Federation on Ageing, Autumn 1979, 6(3), 23.)

The author presents in tables and figures suicide data from the
World Health Organization (primarily for 1970–1972) for 33 more
developed nations. From these patterns Jedlicka suggests there
are three distinct patterns of suicide rates in old age. In
Western countries the rates increase in old age for men while
women exhibit level or falling rates after menopause. In East
European countries male and female   rates   show   "parallel
fluctuations" and the gap between the sexes remains wide in old
age (though smaller than seen in Western countries).   In more
developed Asian countries rates of suicide accelerate greatly
between 50 and 60 years of age for both sexes and the gap
between men and women lessens with increasing old age. The
author's explanation of these differences is that in East
European and Asian countries suicide in old age is related to
rapid social change whereas in Western countries adaptation
rates and the differential ages at which it begins for the sexes
are cited. Earlier adaptation to old age in Western cultures is
triggered by the social significance of menopause and youthful
appearance. Women therefore must perceive themselves as old and
adapt to old age sooner than males, which leads to earlier
suicide peaks and lessening of rates as adaptation takes place.
The abrupt change and need for adaptation for males as they move
from great activity to passivity is felt to lead to hopelessness
and suicide. In Asian and East European countries youth is less
valued than it is in the West while respect for ancestry, mutual
dependence, etc., are valued highly.   Therefore, forces to
suicide more equally affect both sexes. The great social change
in these countries is used to explain the rate increases in old

age for both sexes.

4-036   Kastenbaum, Robert, & Mishara, Brian L. (1971, July).   Premature
        death and self-injurious behavior in old age.   Geriatrics, 26,
        71-81.

        This paper is concerned with the concept of premature death in
        old age.   After discussing several   possible   meanings   of
        premature death and comparing the concept to premature birth of
        babies, the authors suggest that all avoidable deaths are
        premature. A discussion of overt suicide as one form of
        premature death follows. The fact that the old commit suicide
        more often than any other age group is noted.

        Subintentional suicide is discussed as another form of premature
        death. The person who increases the probability of his own
        demise without conscious knowledge of this disposition or who
        uses methods that are indirect may be classified as having a
        subintentioned suicidal orientation.   The psychological autopsy
        may be used to determine, after the fact, how large a role the
        individual played in his or her own death.

        Kastenbaum and Mishara report the findings of a study of 64 male
        and 142 female nonpsychiatric inpatients at a state mental
        hospital. The mean ages of the men and women were 70.3 and 72
        years, respectively.   The study examined the incidence   of
        self-injurious behavior of elderly patients institutionalized
        for chronic, irreversible medical problems.   Charge attendants
        recorded all self-injurious behaviors (SIB) observed during a
        7-day period. Unfortunately, no control group was chosen with
        which to compare results. The findings showed a very high level
        of self-injurious behaviors for the patients studied.   Such
        behaviors were observed at least once in 43.8% of the men and
        21.8% of the women. Men were more likely to engage in SIB than
        were women in the sample. A discussion of five major forms of
        SIB is included.   Among those SIB forms discussed are refusing
        medication, smoking or drinking against medical advice, and
        failing to follow medical orders.

        The final section of the paper offers some implications for
        physicians. The emphasis is on adequate recognition   and
        assessment of subtle suicidal symptoms.

4-037   Kessel, Neil. (1967). Self-poisoning.   In Edwin S. Shneidman
        (Ed.), Essays in self-destruction (pp. 344-372).   New York:
        Science House. (Condensed from British Medical Journal, 1965,
        Issue 5473, pp. 1264-1270 & 1965, Issue 5474, pp. 1336-1348.)

        This general article on self-poisoning (a term used instead of
        attempted suicide) includes a consideration of age differences.
        Data by age presented for Edinburgh indicate that for males,
        rates of self-poisoning are low in teenage years (20-25 per
        100,000 population), higher and stable from 20-65 years of age
        (rate=80-100), and very low over age 65 (rates less than 25).

For females, rates are very high among the young (rate for 20–25 year olds=280) and rates decline regularly with increasing age such that above 45 years of age there are no differences between the sexes (i.e., very low rates in old age for females also). While the young frequently employed salicylates, the use of barbiturates and coal gas rose with age. This was explained as a result of availablity. The young have less insomnia and therefore less availability than the old to sleeping pills (so they turn instead to an available drug, salicylates). The old, it is suggested, more often use coal gas because they are alone long enough to die from this method and presumably there are no young children in the house to be endangered by the use of this method. "Cultural factors may also be important; when they were younger it [coal gas] was one of the traditional methods of self-poisoning [in Edinburgh], and they have carried this accepted pattern with them into old age. The young people of today probably will not employ gassing when they get old" (p. 356).

4-038   Kiorboe, Erik. (1951). Suicide and attempted suicide among old people. Journal of Gerontology, 6, 233–236.

This study presents data for the suicidal behavior among institutionalized elderly in De Gamles By of Copenhagen from 1933 to 1948. All cases of suicide (N=14, all males) and "the most serious" suicide attempts (N=21; 11 males, 10 females) were included. Almost all individual cases had lived in the institution for 3 or more years. Motives to suicide for this group include recurrent acute physical pain often accompanied by depression for completers and physical illness or disease and often depression for attempters. Mental illness was present in all but 2 of the 35 cases. Alcoholism was a factor in 5 of the completers but none of the attempters. None of the completers, but 11 of the attempters showed symptoms of dementia. Violent methods (usually hanging, stangulation, or jumping from heights) were used among all attempters and by 12 of 14 completers. One completer each employed gas and drugs. The choice of violent methods rather than drugs was "probably [due to] the lack of sufficient energy or ingenuity to obtain poisons" (p. 235) or the presence of dementia may have been a factor in the choice. The absence of dementia among completed suicides, but their prevalence among attempters (11 of 21) suggests that "a debilitated constitution may aggravate an existing dementia and provoke an attempt at suicide, which is seldom successful because of mental and physical weakness" (p. 235). Among these institutionalized elders, marital conflicts, financial problems, and loneliness were rare as motives for suicide. The small number of cases on which these data are based should be kept in mind, the criteria for inclusion as a "serious attempt" was not stated, and it seems fairly clear from the information that those who commit suicide and those who attempt may represent different populations of institutionalized elderly.

4-039   Kivela, Sirkka-Liisa. (1985). Relationship between suicide, homicide and accidental deaths among the aged in Finland in 1951-1979. Acta Psychiatrica Scandinavica, 72, 154-160.

The author presents trends in official data over time (1951-1979) for suicide, homicide, and accidental deaths among the aged (65+) of Finland. While small fluctuations occurred, the suicide rates overall and for both sexes could best be described as exhibiting little change over the period of study. In an attempt to discover whether homicide and accidents reflect self-destructive tendencies among the elderly as in suicide, correlation coefficients were computed between the mortality rates for these causes and suicide. Significant correlations with suicide mortality were found only among elderly males for motor vehicle accidents (r=.53, p<.01) and total accidents (r=.64, p<.001). No significant relations were seen among elderly females. The author concluded that "self-destructiveness may play some role in motor-vehicle accident mortality among the aged male population" (p. 160) but it is not important in elderly female accident mortality Methodological problems of the investigation are noted.

4-040 Klein-Schwartz, Wendy, Oderda, Gary M., & Booze, Lisa. (1983). Poisoning in the elderly. Journal of the American Geriatrics Society, 31, 194-199.

This study investigated the nature and incidence of poisoning in elderly callers to the Maryland Poison Control Center. All calls during a six month period involving patients 60 years and older were examined. The final study group consisted of 237 patients ranging in age from 60 to 97. The sample was comprised of 66% females. The majority of calls were received from non-medical personnel, mostly relatives or friends. The major location of the poisoning was the home and the primary route of the exposure was oral. Of the total cases, 197 were classified as accidents, 35 as suicide attempts, and 7 as drug abuse. Of the 4 deaths, 3 were suicides. The major reasons accidental poisonings occurred were senility and confusion, improper use or storage of a product, or mistaken identities of products. The authors call for more education efforts aimed at preventing accidental poisoning in the elderly population.

4-041 Kockott, Gotz. (1979). Suicidal behaviour in the elderly: Relevant sociodemographic variables in comparison to a younger suicidal population. In H. Orimo, K. Shimada, M. Iriki, & D. Maeda (Eds.), Recent advances in gerontology (pp. 181-182). Amsterdam: Excerpta Medica.

A brief presentation is made of an investigation into sociodemographic variable (sex, marital status) differences between two suicide attempter populations and the population as a whole in the Federal Republic of Germany. The two suicide attempter populations were 4010 patients below the age of 65 and 180 who were 65 years of age or above. These attempters had been seen as patients at a psychiatric institute between 1970

and 1976 as a result of their attempt. Among the younger
attempters, higher ratios of females than males were seen when
compared to the normal population. Comparable sex ratios to
those of the normal population were found among elderly
attempters however. For suicide attempts, therefore, elderly
males seem to be as much at risk as females. Among both young
and older attempter groups divorced individuals were
overrepresented while the married were underrepresented. The
ratio of widowed patients was consistent with that in the
general population for both age groups of attempters. While the
divorced and widowed share the loss of a partner, the above
results are explained "partly in the nature of the suicide
attempt as an appeal directed mainly at the still-existing but
divorced partner" (p. 182). Among older attempters higher
proportions of depressive diagnoses were seen than for the young
(46% vs. 30%), whereas higher ratios among the young were found
for diagnoses of schizophrenia, alcoholism, drug addiction, and
transient situational disturbances. Both younger and older
attempters shared most frequently the motives of conflict with
partners for their suicide attempt as well as conflict with
other relatives and social isolation. Concern about illness
(10%) and fear of changing life circumstances (4%) were also
motives seen among the older attempters. The latter concerns,
especially about physical illness, are more common among elderly
completed suicides (according to the literature) whereas
interpersonal conflicts are seen most often for attempters.

4-042   Kruijt, C. S. (1977). The suicide rate in the Western world
since World War II. Netherlands Journal of Sociology, 13,
54-64.

This article presents official World Health Organization data
(especially for 1947-1969) for a number of European countries
and employs social phenomena as a major explanation of suicide
rates generally, by sex and age, and especially among the aged.
Kruijt notes first that suicide rates for Central Western
European and other Anglo-Saxon cultures (e.g., U.S.A., Canada,
Australia, New Zealand) were stable or declined after the turn
of the century and to WWII. The outlying Northern and Southern
European countries, on the other hand, displayed increasing
suicide rates at that time. The explanation given is that the
stress and necessity to cope with rapid changes associated with
industrialization took place prior to or soon after 1900 for the
former countries but took place later in the century for the
latter nations; thus, the varying suicide rates associated with
temporal industrialization variations. Rates among women were
suggested to be rising while those for men were decreasing or
stable, again as a result of differential effects of
industrialization. However, with "female emancipation" this
protected position is increasingly lessened and women are
exposed to negative social aspects to which men to some extent
have become acclimated.

Following WWII, the focus of the paper, women's rates continued to rise but the rates for men in many countries did not continue to be stable or decline but rather increased. Following logical discussions of potential contributing factors, the author dismisses chance fluctuations in rates and economic factors as explanations for the increased male rates. Looking at changes in the data presented by age for males from the late 1940s to late 1960s, Kruijt observes the increase for the young age groups (especially 24-34), a decrease for the 65-74 male age group that was not present in earlier data, while most other age groups were little changed. Therefore, the increased male rates were largely the result of increases for adolescent and young adult males. Declines for males 64-74 "may tend to counter this, but it is not numerically large enough to compensate for the influence that the increase among young people has on the total rate" (p. 60). Kruijt calls the decline in 64-74 male suicide rates "the most striking phenomenon in the post-war development of the specific suicide rates" (p. 60). His suggested explanation for this decline is the concomitant large and rapid improvement in the circumstances and position of the old after WWII. The decline begins from 1956-1965, at the same time as extremely rapid growth for the countries discussed. As a part of overall growth, the amount of money spent on welfare and health services for the aged also took place. Women over the age of 45 and particularly 64-74 have shown increases during this time period. While women have also shared the greater economic and social security as well as medical and social benefits of increased prosperity, countering factors have apparently had a greater effect. However, Kruijt makes no attempt to suggest what these factors might be. Another explanation contributing to declining elderly male rates that the author suggests is changing attitudes toward retirement. These changing attitudes involve viewing retirement as a welcomed life period rather than one of frustration and loss (women's roles have not usually involved such an abrupt change at the traditional age of retirement and this may be a patial explanation for their not sharing in decreased rates). No reduction in suicide rates was seen for males over 75 and Kruijt suggests that such individuals have not shared in some of the benefits of the younger cohorts, especially in a psychological fashion, and also this period of life is one of increased physical decline. Finally, a general explanation for the lack of sharing decreased rates exhibited by young-old males among 75+ males and aged women is that "the direct influence of social factors decreases the less one participates in social life" (p. 64). Interestingly, Kruijt says nothing about increased rates for young males other than noting that they took place.

4-043 Leenaars, Antoon A., & Balance, William D. G. (1984). A predictive approach to suicide notes of young and old people from Freud's formulations with regard to suicide. Journal of Clinical Psychology, 40, 1362-1364.

This study examined suicide notes written by 52 individuals of various ages (range=18-74 years). Based on specific statements

about suicide made by Sigmund Freud throughout his writings, 25
protocol statements were derived. Two independent judges
(clinicians with graduate degrees in psychology) were asked to
read the 52 letters and determine whether each contained content
that was reflected by the individual 25 protocol statements. No
demographic or other information about the note writers was
provided to the judges; only the notes were given to them.
High interjudge reliability was found for the classifications
with respect to the protocol statements. The content of the
protocol statements was found more frequently in the notes of
young people ("young" defined as below the mean age of the note
writers, i.e., 42 years; "old" defined as above the mean age of
42). The only significant differences between younger and older
letter writers' content involved the presence of several themes
more often in the letters of younger writers: communication of
a sense of guilt or criticism, feelings of extreme harshness and
severity toward oneself, and feelings that they must kill
themselves because they deserve no better fate. Overall, there
were many more similarities between the notes than there were
differences. Particularly common descriptions in the notes of
both young and old were: conscious choice regarding the time,
method and opportunity for their death; conscious planning of
the suicide act although motivations are apparently unconscious;
and loss or rejection of a significant other.   The authors
conclude that "age is a significant variable when one is
examining the dynamics of the suicidal person" (p. 1363).   The
findings are in general agreement with those of Farberow and
Shneidman (1957/1970, reference 4-024) and Lester and Hummel
(1980, reference 4-049) with regard to less inwardly-directed
aggression expressed by the old than young in their notes.
[Note: The suicide notes were provided by David Lester and
apparently are the same ones utilized by Lester & Hummel, 1980,
reference 4-049, and Lester & Reeve, 1982, reference 4-050.]

4-044 Lester, David. (1971). MMPI scores of old and young completed
       suicides. Psychological Reports, 28, 146.

       The MMPI (Minnesota Multiphasic Personality Inventory) scores of
       52 white hospitalized males were correlated with their age
       (range 14-81 years; mean age=34 years; only 5 subjects were
       above 50 however). Significant correlations for age and several
       MMPI subscores were observed.   The old "showed significantly
       more response conformity (F scale), . . . less denial of
       personal inadequacies (K scale). . . . less often use physical
       symptoms as a means of resolving conflicts (Hy scale) and a
       greater tendency to paranoia (Pa scale)." The old had no higher
       scores than the young on scales tapping psychotic and neurotic
       processes however.

4-045 Lester, David. (1973). Suicide, homicide, and age-dependency
       ratios. International Journal of Aging and Human Development,
       4, 127-132.

       Utilizing two age-dependency ratios (ratio of those under 15 to those 14–64, and the ratio of those over 65 to those 15–64), Lester compares 28 nations on the incidence of homicide and suicide. Spearman rank correlation coefficients were computed and Lester reports that higher proportions of young dependents were associated with higher homicide and lower suicide rates. Conversely, larger proportions of old dependents were associated with higher suicide and lower homicide rates. Lester hypothesized that stresses in societies with a large proportion of young people lead to the acting–out of aggression (higher homicide rates), while stresses in societies with a larger proportion of older people lead to the internalization of aggression (higher suicide rates).

4–046   Lester, David. (1982). The distribution of sex and age among completed suicides: A cross-national study. International Journal of Social Psychiatry, 28, 256–260.

The idea for this paper was based on statements attributed to Fuse in a 1980 work (the specific reference is not given). Fuse had suggested three descriptive patterns of suicide rates by age in various cultures: (1) regular increases with age, (2) bimodal with a lesser peak in young adulthood and a larger one in old age, and (3) one that peaks in middle age (an inverted U–shaped curve). Fuse had hypothesized that in East–Asian countries females represent a higher proportion of suicides and that bimodal patterns of suicide rates by age are characteristic of developing nations. To test the validity of these age patterns and the two hypotheses, Lester obtained World Health Organization data for 1975 for a number of nations. He found that Asian countries indeed had significantly lower male:female ratios of suicide rates than did European and South American/Middle American/Carribean nations. Fuse's three age pattern categories were not supported well and the bimodal pattern was not exclusive to or necessarily found in developing nations (developing as measured by the gross national product per capita [GNP]). Economic activity based on this GNP measure was significantly related to the age distribution but only for females. Three pages of tables are presented with data and pattern characterizations by age and sex for various nations.

4–047   Lester, David. (1984). Suicide risk by birth cohort. Suicide and Life–Threatening Behavior, 14, 132–136.

Suicide risk was studied among U.S. male and female 5–year birth cohorts, represented by official suicide rates by age at 5–year intervals beginning with 1935 (to 1975). Using such 5–year data, the suicide rates of birth cohorts may be followed as the cohort ages through time. Lester found that female birth cohorts with high suicide rates at earlier life periods had lower rates 14–25 years later and conversely, those with low suicide rates at earlier life periods had higher rates 14–25 years later. For males, however, data indicated that birth cohorts had similar rates at all points in their life so that if the rates were high at younger ages they were high also at older ages. Different suicide patterns by birth cohort were therefore observed for the sexes. Lester states that at present there are no apparent explanations for these sex differences for birth cohorts.

4-048   Lester, David, & Beck, Aaron T. (1974).   Age differences in patterns of attempted suicide. Omega: Journal of Death and Dying, 5, 317-322.

An investigation of 246 attempted suicides seen at a general hospital is presented.   An attempter under 10 years of age was excluded leaving 245 attempters distributed as follows by age: 31 who were 10-19 years of age; 117, 56, 26, and 15, who were 20-29, 30-39, 40-49, and 50 or above, respectively.   Over 50 variables were available for these individuals as a result of interviews conducted as soon after admission as possible.   The variables could be grouped into demographic variables, circumstances of the attempt, precipitating circumstances, physical and psychiatric status, personal history, and psychological tests that were administered. Only 13 significant differences by age were observed. Among these, (1) the proportion of blacks was much lower among attempters aged 50 and above (proportion around 50% for all groups younger than 50; only 7% for 50 and above), (2) the proportion of those living alone increased with age (nearly 50% for those 50+ but 21% or less for groups under 50), (3) the old had fewer in good physical health, (4) although the medical lethality of the attempt for the old did not differ from that of the young more of the old reported an intent to die (100% in those 50+), (5) fewer of the old had made a previous attempt(s) (13% for 50+; percentages 58-73% for younger age groupings), (6) none of the old had recent legal problems, (7) the old (and all age groups above 20) more often abused alcohol (but the old were not more likely to be intoxicated at the time of their attempt) while the young most often abused other drugs, (8) the old were less likely to have a friend(s) tell them that the attempter was in need of help (21% for 50+ compared to 37-60% for other ages), (9) the old and the youngest age groups attempted suicide more often in the winter, and (10) fewer of the old had had a separation from their father in childhood (13% for the old compared to 20-46% of the younger attempters).   No differences between age groups were observed for lethality of the attempt, depression scores, hopelessness scores, suicidal intent, post-attempt suicidal ideation, or severity of mental disturbance. In addition no "shift from interpersonal to intrapsychic factors with increasing age" was found (p. 321). The fewer previous attempts by the old were interpreted such that they had turned to suicide for the first time in old age and did not represent those with "suicidal careers." The small number of elderly (defined as 50 and above, N=15), and the obviously even smaller number above 60 (or older ages) suggests that caution should be taken regarding the results and their generalization to more traditionally defined elderly groupings.

4-049   Lester, David, & Hummel, Holly. (1980).   Motives for suicide   in
elderly people. Psychological Reports, 47, 870.

Ratings (on a seven-point scale) of the motivation (as described
by Menninger, 1938, Man against Himself, New York: Harcourt
Brace) of the writer in 52 suicide notes from police files were
determined by two Ph.D. psychologists.   Contrary to the findings
of Farberow and Shneidman (1957/1970, reference 4-024 of this
book), the older suicides among the note writers (based on
correlational results) were no less likely than young suicide
note writers to express the desire to kill (outward-directed
aggression) or to die, although they were less likely to express
the desire to be killed (inward-directed aggression).

4-050   Lester, David, & Reeve, Calvin. (1982).   The   suicide   notes   of
young and old people. Psychological Reports, 50, 334.

Content   differences   by   age in the suicide notes of 52
individuals (48 completed suicides and 4 attempted suicides;
mean age=42.2 years;   35 males, 17 females) were examined. The
age of the writers was significantly associated only with the
ratio of verbs of feeling to verbs of action (r=-.41) and how
explicitly suicide was stated as the intention (r=-.33). Higher
ages of the note writers, therefore, were associated with more
concern with feelings than actions and being less explicit about
the suicidal action.   No significant relation to age was
observed for a large number of other content elements (e.g.,
note length as measured by words, thought units, words per
thought unit; number of positive, negative, or neutral units,
etc.). [Note: These are apparently the same notes as utilized
by Leenaars & Balance, 1984, reference 4-043, and Lester &
Hummel, 1980, reference 4-049, in which only 5 notes were
written by individuals 50 years of age or older.]

4-051   Lettieri, Dan J. (1973).   Suicide in the aging: Empirical
prediction of suicidal risk among the aging.   Journal of
Geriatric Psychiatry, 6, 7-42.

This article presents the research on the development of a
suicidal death prediction scale, that is a scale that would
predict the risk of suicidal death for an individual. The scale
was developed from cases on file in the Los Angeles Suicide
Prevention Center. A random selection from these files was made
for those callers who were known to be alive (sample N=530) who
were compared to a sample of 52 callers who were known to be
dead by suicide.   The alive sample was further screened to
eliminate those who were not suicidal at the time they contacted
the suicide prevention center.   This eliminated 65 cases,
leaving an alive group of 465 individuals. This group was known
to be alive at least two years after they had made contact with
the center. From a list of 100 potential variables, repeated
reliability checks resulted in 75 items with high reliability
among 12 raters of a randomly selected 10 cases. A total of 12
clinicians who were associated with the center blindly rated all

465 alive and 52 dead cases on each of the 75 items from the
information in their case folders. Stepwise discrimination
function analysis produced high weightings for age and sex.
Therefore, the subject sample was split into four age by sex
groupings as follows: (1) males over 40 years of age (alive
N=59; dead N=17), (2) males under 40 years of age (alive N=115;
dead N=13), (3) females over 40 (alive N=80; dead N=11), and
(4) females under 40 (alive N=211; dead N=11). The analyses
were repeated and resulted in four forms of the scale, each
specific to the characteristics of the individual about which a
suicide death prediction will be made. The analyses also
yielded short and long forms of each scale. The use of these
scales, as described on page 14, is for the worker on a crisis
or suicide prevention telephone service who must assess the
likelihood of suicide among the person who is calling. The long
and short forms of the scales are included in an appendix to the
article along with instructions for their use. The author
emphasizes that the items on the scales were chosen
statistically and not clinically.

4-052   Lonnqvist, Jouko, & Achte, Kalle. (1985). Follow-up study of
the attempted suicides among the elderly in Helsinki in
1973-1979. Crisis: International Journal of Suicide- and
Crisis-Studies, 6, 10-18.

A total of 3040 persons who made 3267 consecutive attempts
resulting in admission to emergency wards of the Helsinki
University General Hospital and directed to psychiatric
consultation from 1933-1979 was studied and followed-up at the
end of 1980. All persons (or their fate) were obtainable at the
follow-up time. Among these 3040 persons, 55 (36 women, 19 men)
were 65 years of age or above (1.8% of total). Structured
interviews were conducted while hospitalized which revealed that
fewer of the elderly (34.5%) had been under psychiatric care
previously (50.8% for the rest of the age groups) and the old
had attempted suicide less often (38.2% vs. 46.3%). The
attempts of the old were more often referred for compulsory
psychiatric hospitalization after their attempt, and the old
were also less likely to have received any psychiatric aftercare
(i.e., no treatment).

At the follow-up period, 20 of the 55 elderly (36.4%) had died.
Of these deaths, 1 was by accident, 14 natural causes, and 5 by
suicide (9.1% of all elderly attempters). The proportion of
elderly females who subsequently committed suicide was 5.6%
while the figure was 15.8% for males. The overall proportion of
attempters who committed suicide was 4.9%. All of the elderly
suicides took place within the first year after the initial
attempt (compared to 57.5% for other ages' suicides).
Therefore, the risk during the first follow-up year was 9.1% for
the old compared to 3.0% for the entire sample. The variables
which predicted subsequent suicide best (as determined by an
observed to expected number of suicides ratio) were, in order,
intention of the attempt as serious, lethality of the attempt as

serious, previous psychiatric treatment, previous attempted suicide, being male, widowed marital status, belonging to the lowest social class, and psychiatric hospitalization after the attempt. It is concluded that attempted suicides are, compared to other age groups, rare among the old. They are, however, more serious and the risk of future suicide is higher. Factors which the case studies imply as predisposing to suicide are depression, somatic illness, and social isolation. It should be noted that "this sample does not include the less severe attempts which are treated only in the outpatient department of the general hospital" (p. 11). The sample, therefore, represents the more serious and severe of attempters at all ages, but if the literature is correct, the old are nearly always serious in the intent to die when they attempt suicide. If this is true, the study results are likely to be conservative estimates of the risk of suicide among attempters for the old compared to the young. Brief case descriptions of the 5 elderly attempters who subsequently committed suicide are included in an appendix.

4-053   Luke, Elizabeth, Norton, William, & Denbigh, Kathryn. (1982). Prevalence of psychologic impairment in an advanced-age population. Journal of the American Geriatrics Society, 30, 114-122.

A sample of 200 individuals aged 80 and above was interviewed in their British Columbia homes. Self-reported psychologic impairment ranged from 14-27% of the sample. Among the psychologically impaired, compared to those who were not, there were lower levels of social contacts and interaction (i.e., isolation) and poorer physical health. Among the information included in the interviews was suicidal ideation ("Have you ever felt so upset that you thought about ending it all?). There were 9 individuals (4.5%) who responded that they had thought about ending it all in the last three years. The proportions were 5.6% among the aged women and 2.7% for the men. These levels may be compared to "less than one-tenth" (Lowenthal & Berkman, 1967, Aging and Mental Disorders in San Francisco, San Francisco: Jossey-Bass), 5% (Kutner, Fanshel, Togo, et al., 1956, Five Hundred Over Sixty: A Community Survey of Aging, New York: Russell Sage), and 2% (Abrahams & Patterson, 1978-79, reference 4-002) in other studies. The authors suggest that "planned programs are needed to improve the lifestyles of the aged and to prevent loneliness and isolation" (p. 114).

4-054   Lyons, Michael J. (1985). Observable and subjective factors associated with attempted suicide in later life. Suicide and Life-Threatening Behavior, 15, 168-183.

The goal of this study was to identify risk factors that differentiate suicide attempters in late life (over 50) from a control group (also over 50). A "retrospective case-control method" was employed in which 118 white control subjects and 34 white attempters were interviewed. The control group was a subset (it is not clear if they were all individuals who were 50 and above, a selected subset, those who would consent to be interviewed, etc. The first criteria seems most likely, however.) of 1847 noninstitutionalized individuals from a random, stratified sample of those living in Northern Kentucky (mean age of the 50 and above group=61.9 years). The attempters consisted of a subset of 113 individuals 50 years and above who had attempted suicide and were identified through emergency room contacts and consultation/liaison psychiatry records over a two and one-half year period. The 34 respondents (mean age=60.4) from among the attempters represented those of the 113 who could be found, were alive, not "too ill," and consented to be interviewed. The Kentucky Social Service Needs Assessment was administered to all subjects in their homes. This questionnaire included measures of socioeconomic status (SES), self-reported ease of availability of social services/mental health services, the extent and quantity of the relational system, positive and negative affect, and perceived life quality/satisfaction. Multiple discriminant analysis was used to determine variables that discriminate between attempters and controls. The final equation correctly classified 81.7% of the sample. The strongest predictor of membership in the attempter group was personal satisfaction (evaluation of themselves), with attempters being less satisfied with/having a more negative evaluation of themselves than the control group. Among the variables associated with attempter group membership were lower SES, expressing less positive and more negative affect, low financial satisfaction, and belonging to fewer organizations (e.g., 56% of the attempter group belonged to no organization compared to 26% of the controls). The author suggests that the retrospective nature of the investigation makes the reliability of the data uncertain. That is, the responses may reflect feelings and conditions prior to, since, or as a consequence of the attempt and not simply prior to the attempt. Another difficulty for this study is that the age inclusion (50 and up) and mean of the sample (60.4 years) suggest the inclusion of few traditionally "old" individuals, and the small number of attempters (N=34) makes this even more problematic for generalization to elderly attempters.

4-055 MacDonald, A. J. D., & Dunn, G. (1982). Death and the expressed wish to die in the elderly: An outcome study. Age and Ageing, 11, 189-195.

Among the continuum of self-destructive behaviors is a group of less direct behaviors called "subintentional" or "indirect self-destructive behaviors." Such behavior involves a varying role on the part of the individual in their own death that may be physical and/or psychological in nature. Expressing the wish to die may in some cases be an example of such behavior. This study resulted from the preliminary screening of older adults 74-89 years of age in London for a study of the frail elderly in different types of care (in-patient wards, day hospitals, day centers, local authority homes). Staff in these facilities were asked to classify attenders or residents of those ages on the degree of dependency on others. Of the attenders, 633 were to some degree personally dependent on others, however, 199 could not provide enough information in an interview and 37 more were discharged before they could be interviewed, leaving 397 individuals in the final sample. A number of factors were tapped in a semistructured interview. As part of a depression scale, subjects were asked "In the past month have you at any time felt you would rather be dead?". Responses were "no", "yes, but rejected suicide", "yes," with suicidal feelings of varying levels, and "yes, attempted suicide". One year later information on the subjects' status (including alive or dead) was obtained from informants at the facilities or other sources. Of the 397 individuals, 65 (16.4%) had died by the one year follow-up (the cause of death was not, however, reported). Discriminant functional analyses revealed that sex, organic brain syndrome scale scores, and the reported wish to die independently predicted membership in the dead or alive category. Those who had died were most often men, with high organic brain syndrome scores, who reported the wish to die. The problems with the study methodology are noted and caution is suggested in interpreting the results.

4-056   MacMahon, Brian, & Pugh, Thomas F. (1965). Suicide in the widowed. American Journal of Epidemiology, 81, 23-31.

This study was conducted to determine whether suicide vs. other causes of death among the widowed differentially cluster in time following the death of their spouse. That is, is bereavement a significant etiological factor. The initial study involved all suicide deaths (N=321) in Massachusetts from 1948-1952 for which the death certificate listed widowed as the marital status of the deceased. A comparison death matched for age, sex, race, and selected for its closeness to the date of the suicide death was chosen for each suicide from among widowed individuals who died from other causes. Such matches were found for 320 of the suicides. Death certificates for the 640 spouses listed on the death certificate of the suicide or matched control subject were then searched for and found for 253 of the 320 suicide deaths (79.1%) and 261 of the 320 comparison deaths (81.6%). Seven of the suicides and their matched controls were eliminated because the widowed person's death was homicide by their spouse, who then committed suicide. The time interval between the deaths of the spouses was calculated for the suicide and comparison groups and it was found that suicide risk (compared to risk of death via other causes) was greater during the first 4 years of widowhood than after and particularly so during the first year. This clustering was even more apparent in older age groups, and particularly among males. The authors argue further that the estimates of the risk differences are likely to be low. Relative risk of suicide for each period was quantified and was indicated to be 2.5 times higher during the first year than the risk four or more years after the death, and 1.5 times higher during the second and third years. Other mathematical manipulations suggested that nearly half (48/109) of the suicides in the first 3 years can be attributed to bereavement. Further comparisons of the suicide group with other comparison groups suggested that it is unlikely that the differential suicide risk can be attributed to the suicidal widowed being less likely to remarry than the less suicidally inclined. Some evidence for higher suicide risk among the widowed of suicides was also presented. The results of this study emphasize the widowed as a high risk population particularly during the first year after their spouses' death. This is especially relevant to the old and middle aged because they comprise the highest risk group for widowhood and these study results suggest the elderly widowers are especially high risk.

4-057   Maris, Ronald. (1985). The adolescent suicide problem. Suicide and Life-Threatening Behavior, 15, 91-109.

As the title of this article implies, this article focuses predominantly on the increase in suicide rates among the young 14-24 since the 1960s. With respect to the old, Maris presents data for a variety of countries by sex and age for 1963-1966 and includes 64-74 and 75+ groupings. He also notes that suicide among older age groupings have been declining and that generally, suicide rates by age seem to be converging to the overall mean (currently approximately 12 per 100,000 population). Maris also reanalyzes the data on which most of his 1981 book Pathways to Suicide (Baltimore: Johns Hopkins University Press) was based. From the sample in that book he selected a representative sample of 266 Chicago suicides based on information from interviews with informants (relatives). He focuses his attention here on how the young (those in their teens and twenties; N=36) differ from and are similar to "older" suicides. The term "older" is not defined and may mean 30 and above or some other more traditional definition of "old." Some caution to generalizations to the over 60 or over 65 population might be taken therefore regarding the statements for "older" suicides. Among the similarities for young and older suicides are: high levels of depression and hopelessness, the use of guns to kill themselves, social isolation, and perceiving death as the only escape from life's problems. Young suicides differ from older suicides in a number of ways, including for the young "more revenge motivated, anger, irritation, and impulsivity-based, have more negative interpersonal relations, make more nonfatal attempts, have more suicides and divorce in their families of origin, are less likely to have financial, work, or marital resources, involve more risk-taking, excessive drug and alcohol use, are more likely to be romantic and idealistic, have lower self-esteem, and fewer life accomplishments" (p. 108).

4-058   Marshall, James R. (1978). Changes in aged white male suicide: 1948-1972. Journal of Gerontology, 33, 763-768.

The annual U.S. official suicide rates for white males 64-74

years of age compared to similarly aged white females were
compiled and contributing factors to the trends were studied.
The trends revealed declines for males but stability for females
over the period of study (1947-1972). The 1972 male suicide
rate was less than 60% that for 1947. In an attempt to explain
the declines in elderly white male suicide, Marshall gathered
data over the same time period for: the unemployment rate of
aged males, those aged males 65 and above who have an income,
the proportion of the labor force that is covered by Social
Security, and the average monthly husband-wife Social Security
payment (adjusted for inflation). The zero-order correlation
for each of the three economic measures to the elderly white
male suicide rates was "strong and negative" (p. 765;
correlations ranged from -.80 to -.93). Unemployment was
positively (r=.40) related to the suicide rate. A multivariate
analysis was also conducted in which a model included a measure
of social cohesion (divorce rate), economic conditions
(unemployment and one of the three indicators of income status
listed above), war (as a dummy variable), and which took into
effect "the time-series dynamics of suicide" (p. 766). The
model accounted for most of the variance in the suicide rate and
found that changes in income status among aged white males was
highly and negatively related to their suicide rates (and
therefore, the declines). The effect was the same regardless of
which of the three economic indicators above were included in
the model. None of the other variables, including unemployment,
were significant. The decline therefore in elderly white male
suicides has been significantly influenced by economic condition
increases but not by the social and political conditions
included here.

4-059   McIntosh, John L. (1984). Components of the decline in elderly
suicide: Suicide among the young-old and old-old by race and
sex. Death Education, 8(Supplement), 113-124.

Official U.S. suicide statistics by sex and race (white
vs. nonwhite) were compiled from 1933 to 1978 for the 54-74, 65
and above, 75 and above, and 85 and above age groupings as well
as 5- and 10-year age groups above 55. The focus of the study
was on demographic groups which had contributed to the declines
in elderly suicide. For the 65 and older population, suicide
rates had declined for both sexes but particularly for males.
Declines were seen among white elderly but nonwhite elderly
rates remained stable. Within the 65+ population, all age
groupings displayed declines but virtually all of the decline
can be seen for males and whites in each age grouping. Among
males and whites, rates for the old-old (75+) declined markedly
but somewhat less than for the young-old (64-74 or 54-74).
Within the old-old population, the declines have been greater
for 74-84 males than for those 85+. Explanations for declines
in elderly suicide are discussed, including economic factors,
the increasing number of women (a low risk group for suicide) in
the elderly population, and cohort differences. Further
research to explain declines in elderly suicide are needed.

4-060   McIntosh, John L. (1985). Suicide among the elderly: Levels and trends.   American   Journal of Orthopsychiatry, 55, 288-293.

Official U.S. data are presented for elderly (65+) suicide from 1900-1980 and in more detail for 1978 for age, sex, and race. The data demonstrate that the elderly are at highest risk for suicide by age (despite the recent attention given to increased youth suicide) and that the rates have declined dramatically for the old. The old commit a disproportionate number of suicides and according to the literature make many fewer and more serious attempts than do the young. Clues to suicide and prevention are briefly discussed. The need for public education regarding suicide clues, community resource availability, and about the aged and suicide in general are highlighted.

4-061   McIntosh, John L., Hubbard, Richard W., & Santos, John F. (1985). Suicide facts and myths: A study of prevalence. Death Studies, 9, 267-281.

Batchelor (1957, reference 3-003, p. 143) begins a chapter on "Suicide in old age," by stating that "If the layman were asked to guess if suicide is common in old age, probably he would answer no. Old people, he might argue, are not given to rash and violent actions but are typically overcautious and conservative, and he would remember the many old people he had known who had clung so tenaciously to the tatters of their lives." The study by McIntosh et al. attempts to determine what the "layperson" (or at least the college students among them) might say if asked such questions. As a first study of this, 271 college students in South Bend, IN were asked 32 factual questions about suicide. In general, information levels were low (Mean=59.1%, or 18.9 items correctly answered out of 32). Among the questions were two that are particularly relevant here. Nearly all (96%) of the respondents knew that suicide rates were increasing among the young, but only 29% correctly responded "False" to a statement that suicide rates among the young were higher than among the old. Therefore, most respondents did not know that the old are a high-risk group for suicide and Batchelor's suggestion is supported. Detailed information on the other questions asked are provided. The authors suggest that suicide is a major mental health problem and that education about high risk groups is needed to aid recognition of suicides as well as prevention and intervention efforts.

4-062   McIntosh, John L., & Santos, John F. (1981). Suicide among minority elderly: A preliminary investigation. Suicide and Life-Threatening Behavior, 11, 151-166.

Official U.S. suicide statistics are compiled for specific racial/ethnic minorities by age for the year 1976 compared to 1959-61 (the latter presented in Morton Kramer, Earl S. Pollack, Richard Redick, & Ben Z. Locke, 1972, Mental Disorders/Suicide, Cambridge, MA: Harvard University Press, p. 179). Data are combined with population estimates to calculate rates by age and sex for blacks, Native Americans (American Indians), Chinese-, Japanese-, and Filipino-/Pilipino Americans compared with whites. Heterogeneity rather than homogeneity was observed among these minorities and their elderly. Overall, Native Americans in 1976 had the highest rates of suicide, followed in descending order of rates by whites, Chinese-Americans, Japanese-Americans, blacks, and Filipino-Americans. By age, suicide rates were highest among the young and very low among the elderly for Native Americans and blacks. Age patterns for whites and all three other Asian-American groups, on the other hand, increased with age, peaking in old age. Filipino-American rates of suicide were highest in old age but their rates were relatively low at all ages. In descending order by 1976 rates, elderly suicide was highest among Chinese-Americans, followed by Japanese-Americans, whites, Filipino-Americans, blacks and Native Americans. Although still high, the suicide rates for both Chinese- and Japanese-American elderly had declined dramatically from the earlier 1959-61 data. A similar but much less pronounced decline was seen for white elderly as well. Little change from earlier levels of suicide was observed for elderly blacks and Native Americans, however youth suicide rates had increased noticeably for both minorities as they had also for whites. Explanations for the differential rates are suggested. Particularly highlighted is the dying out of the sojourner generations among Chinese- and Japanese-American elderly to account for the large declines in suicide seen for their aged. The "survivor" status of aged blacks and Native Americans as well as life-long adaptation to low status (i.e., old age is not an abrupt change as is often is for whites, especially for white males) are discussed as possible reasons for low rates in these elderly. The need for long-term data and figures for Hispanics are noted. The former are reported for the same minorities for 1968-1981 in a paper entitled Suicide Among Minority Elderly that was presented by McIntosh at the November 1985 meeting of the Gerontological Society of America in New Orleans, LA.

4-063   McIntosh, John L., & Santos, John F. (1985-86). Methods of suicide by age: Sex and race differences among the young and old. International Journal of Aging and Human Development, 22, 123-139.

The literature contains many explanations for the greater likelihood that the old (compared to the young) will die if they attempt suicide. One of the most commonly cited of these is that the old use more lethal methods in their attempts than do the young. Most authors who make this statement provide no data to support the contention however (e.g., Batchelor, 1957, reference 3-003;   Patterson et al., 1974, reference 3-037; Resnik & Cantor, 1970, reference 3-045). While the statement is almost certainly true from the data of attempters, it is uncertain among those who complete suicide. This study compiles annual official U.S. suicide data from 1960 to 1978 by age, sex, and race (white, black, nonwhite excluding black [NWEB]) for the methods of suicide employed. Rates and annual percentages of the total number of suicides for each method individually, for all poisons combined (i.e., "less lethal" methods) and firearms and hanging combined (i.e., "lethal" methods) were calculated. The hypothesis that the old complete suicide more often than the young because they employ more lethal methods was not totally confirmed by these data. While elderly white males, blacks of both sexes, and NWEB females employed more lethal methods than their corresponding young, no age differences in method usage were found for NWEB males, and opposite results were observed among white females (i.e., young white females employed lethal methods more often than elderly white women). Therefore, the differential completion of suicidal acts by the old and young is not wholly explained by method differences (although it is likely to be an important contributing factor). As found in other studies (e.g., McIntosh & Santos, 1982, Changing patterns in methods of suicide by race and sex, Suicide and Life-Threatening Behavior, 12, 221-233), all age-sex-racial groups displayed increased firearm use over time. In fact among women, a group traditionally employing poisons most often for suicide, firearms comprised equal or higher proportions to that of poisons in the last years of data. The problems with aggregate data for the nonwhite population and subgroups such as NWEB are discussed with respect to the resulting disguised differences among specific racial/ethnic groups that comprise the aggregated grouping. The use of more lethal methods by the old among those who die, especially for elderly white males, the highest risk group for suicide overall, underscores the special need for preventive attention. Cohort studies for suicide methods are also suggested.

4-064   Megenhagen, Paula M., Lee, Barrett A., & Gove, Walter R. (1985). Till death do us part: Recent changes in the relationship between marital status and mortality. Sociology and Social Research, 70, 53-56.

These authors compare 1959-61 vs. 1979 U.S. official mortality data for suicide by marital status, sex, and age. The article is almost exclusively a presentation of data with virtually no discussion of the implications or explanations of the findings. Suicide is but one of 11 causes of death for which data are presented for the age groupings 25-44, 45-64, and 65+. No specific suicide rates are given, as the authors present only Marital Status Mortality Ratios (MSWR) which compare the mortality of the never married, widowed, and divorced with that of the married population of the same age and sex. For the elderly (and generally for all age groups as well), the divorced population was at highest risk for suicide but less so than in the earlier 1959-61 data. In 1979 divorced females over 65 had an MSMR of 2.65 which means that their suicide rate was over two and one-half times that for married elderly females. Corresponding MSMRs were 1.62 for widowed elderly females and 1.36 for never married aged females. For elderly males, the

MSMRs were close for the divorced and widowed with the widowed
value actually slightly exceeding that for the divorced (2.66
and 2.58, respectively). Never married elderly males had a
suicide MSMR of 1.96. As can be seen, in all cases married
elders were at lower risk than the other groupings for suicide
(i.e., MSMRs exceeded 1.00) and those with marital disruptions
through widowhood or divorce were at higher risk than those
never married. These patterns are similar to those in the
earlier literature and reflect the high risk status of those
with a loss or disruption in the very important interpersonal
relationship of marriage.

4-065   Miller, Marv. (1978a). Note: Toward a profile of the older
        white male suicide. Gerontologist, 18, 80–82.

This brief article presents a listing of the characteristics
most commonly seen among geriatric suicides studied by Miller or
characteristics seen (statistically) significantly more often in
the geriatric suicides than among a matched control group.
These characteristics are based on 30 older (apparently 60 and
above) white male suicides from among 301 consecutive cases in
Arizona from 1970–1975. Data were derived from interviews with
the surviving widows of the 30 older white men from Maricopa
County, AZ who committed suicide. Generalizability problems
from only 30 cases are recognized by the author, but the
"typical" older white male suicide in this sample included
(among many listed) the following characteristics: was 68 years
old, married, retired, had a current annual income of less than
$5000, lived with a friend or relative at the time of his death,
had a confidant (usually his wife), used a firearm (most often a
pistol) to kill himself, was not an active member of any
organizations (civic, fraternal, religious), had visited a
physician within a month of his suicide, had a serious physical
illness during the year before death, felt inadequate and useless
as well as unhappy and depressed, gave verbal or behavioral
clues to his suicide. In addition, the suicides differed
significantly from the matched controls on these
characteristics: they seldom attended church, had no
visitations with friends or relatives even at least once a week,
left a note for someone, left a will, experienced sleep problems
during the year prior to death, were addicted to drugs, had a
relative with mental or emotional illness, and committed suicide
at home.

4-066   Miller, Marv. (1978b). Geriatric suicide: The Arizona study.
        The Gerontologist, 18, 488–495.

Information on death certificates and personal data obtained
through interviews with surviving family members or friends for
older white male suicides (N=301) occurring in Arizona from 1970
to 1975 were reported. These data revealed that the vast
majority (85%) of these older men employed firearms as their
suicide method. A subset of 30 older white male suicides in one
Arizona county was also studied. The study of these 30 suicides

indicated that the death of the person's confidant was more
likely than among a matched group that had died of natural
causes, and that most (76%) of the elderly suicides had visited
a physician within a month of their death, with one-third
visiting within a week. Most (60%) of these 30 suicides had
given verbal or behavioral clues to their suicide, but some
survivors (23%) had not recognized the clues that were given.
Examples from the 30 suicides but no specific data are presented
for Miller's statement that "It appears that poor planning for,
and poor adjustment to, retirement is a major negative factor in
the suicides of older men in the USA" (p. 495).

4-067   Mishara, Brian L., & Kastenbaum, Robert. (1973). Self-injurious
behavior and environmental change in the institutionalized
elderly. International Journal of Aging and Human Development,
4, 133-145.

The focus of this study was on the effects of the environment on
self-injurious behavior (SIB). The authors explored both a
humanistic and a behavior modification approach to changing the
environment and the effect of each on SIB. Two different
rehabilitation programs were set up for elderly residents of a
medical unit of a large state mental hospital. One consisted of
several humanistic forms of environmental enrichment free to all
residents (the Enrichment Ward). The other set up a system
whereby all enrichments had to be earned by residents engaging
in "desirable behaviors" (the Token Economy).

There were 80 experimental group subjects (40 male, 40 female
selected randomly, with a mean age of 68.8 years) and 55 control
group subjects from the same unit (25 male, 30 female) involved
in the study. Subjects were assigned to the Enrichment Ward or
Token Economy condition for a 9 month period. Observations of
self-injurious behavior were recorded for all participants,
including members of the control group. Results revealed that
SIB was much less frequent on the two treatment wards than on
the control ward. The Token Economy condition showed the least
SIB. The study suggests that the amount of SIB among elderly
mental hospital residents may be decreased by improving the
quality of the environment.

4-068   Modi, Shams-ul-Ulma J. J. (1904-1907). Suicides and old age.
Journal of the Anthropological Society of Bombay, 7, 577-590.

The author responds to a statement by Elie Metchnikoff (in a
1904 report to the Smithsonian Institution) that the old often
kill themselves and at rates higher than for younger ages.
Presenting data for India by age from 1894-1905, Modi shows that
rates overall were very low in comparison to those of Western
societies and that rates among the old were considerably lower
than those for the younger (20-50) population. Modi suggests
that Eastern cultural teaching about respecting and supporting
the elderly is stronger than in the West and customs such as
living in the same household and being advised to marry and have

children (especially sons) increase adherence and teaching of respect and support. This early paper points to the tremendous cultural differences that have, and continue, to exist in elderly suicide, and the likelihood that cultural practices and beliefs influence these levels.

4-069   Murphy, George E., & Wetzel, Richard D. (1980). Suicide risk by birth cohort in the United States, 1949 to 1974. Archives of General Psychiatry, 37, 519-523.

These authors examined official suicide rates for specific birth cohorts by considering data at successive 5-year intervals beginning with 1949. The results were similar to those by Solomon and Hellon (1980, reference 4-094) for Alberta, Canada. Specifically, beginning about 1955, the suicide rate for each successive 5-year birth cohort was higher than the rate of the preceding birth cohort when it was of the same age. This trend is not exclusively noted at young ages, but occurs at older ages as well and among all sex and race groups. These data suggest substantially higher suicide rates in the younger cohorts as they age. While the data presented only allow the birth cohorts since the beginning of the phenomenon to be followed to age 40-44, the implication could clearly be that rates for these cohorts may be higher at older ages as well. Such an effect would be to reverse current declines in rates among middle age and older adults. The need to investigate further using cohort analyses is stated.

4-070   Nelson, Franklyn L. (1977). Religiosity and self-destructive crises in the institutionalized elderly. Suicide and Life-Threatening Behavior, 7, 67-74.

The focus of this study was on the relationship between intensity of religious commitment to the use of indirect life-threatening behavior (ILTB) among elderly, chronically ill hospital patients. A nonrandom sample of 58 intensive care unit patients (mean age=62.2) drawn from the Veterans Administration's Wadsworth Hospital Center in Los Angeles was studied. Patients whose faculties of judgment and reasoning were severely impaired were excluded. The ILTB was measured by a rating scale designed to record the range of observable life-threatening behaviors and provide a relative ranking of patients. Nurses observed and rated patients' behavior 24 hours a day for 7 days, regarding the occurrences of any one or more of 56 life-threatening behaviors (e.g., refusing medications, pulling out I.V. needle). Scale scores ranged from 0 (no ILTB) to 151. Religiosity was measured both in terms of church affiliation and religious commitment. Data on affiliation were obtained from medical records. The patients were interviewed and asked if they subscribed to a particular set of religious teachings and, if so, how important a role these beliefs played in their life. This provided a measure of the intensity of religious commitment.

Findings from the study revealed that the more devout the patient was in his/her religious beliefs, the less likely he/she was to engage in ILTB. The incidence of ILTB did not differ greatly, however, among religious affiliations. Strong religious beliefs nourish feelings of worthfulness and hopefulness, and provide a source of goal-directed behavior involved in following the teachings which serves to reduce feelings of helplessness.

4-071   Nelson, Franklyn L., & Farberow, Norman L. (1977). Indirect suicide in the elderly chronically ill patient. In Kalle Achte & Jouko Lonnqvist (Eds.), Suicide research: Proceedings of the seminars of suicide research by Yrjo Jahnsson Foundation 1974-1977 (pp. 124-139). Helsinki, Finland: Psychiatria Fennica, Psychiatria Fennica Supplementum 1976.

The authors' concern in this study is with indirect forms of self-destruction and the nature and extent of such suicidal behavior among the hospitalized elderly. Indirect life-threatening behavior (ILTB) is defined as any behavior which shortens life and results in premature death. Examples of ILTB include: failure to follow specified medical regimens, alcoholism or drug abuse, and hyperobesity. The study was conducted among patients hospitalized on the intensive care unit of Wadsworth Veterans Administration Hospital Center in Los Angeles. A scale of ILTB was developed (and is included in an appendix) which could be used by nurses and other raters observing behavior of patients. The development of the rating scale is described in the article and the present study included ratings for 58 patients.

Several hypotheses were tested, including: the patient who engages in ILTB will score high on suicide potential; those who engage in ILTB tend to be older and have more medical problems; and those who engage in ILTB are less religious. Patients and staff were interviewed to gather data on social and psychological dimensions. The small sample precluded rigorous statistical analyses but a correlation matrix is presented. The most important correlates of ILTB were the extent of personal loss experienced, satisfaction with hospital life, life satisfaction, orientation towards risk taking, and suicide potential. A pattern of dissatisfaction, loss, and isolation is associated with self-destructive potential.

4-072   Nelson, Franklyn L., & Farberow, Norman L. (1980). Indirect self-destructive behavior in the elderly nursing home patient. Journal of Gerontology, 35, 949-957.

Indirect self-destructive behavior (ISDB) includes such actions as refusing to eat or drink, diet management, failure to follow specified medical regimens, and other behaviors which injure, defeat, distress, and shorten life. The study was conducted on 99 chronically ill white male veteran patients over the age of 65 in seven Veterans Administration nursing homes in the Los

Angeles, CA area. The patients were observed and rated on their
ISDBs over a 13 month period. They were interviewed extensively
to obtain data on physical health, psychological and personality
dimensions (including a measure of suicide risk), factors such
as recent loss, and the availability of social and material
resources.

Data analyses revealed that the highest incidence of ISDB occurs
among patients having a primary diagnosis of diabetes mellitus.
ISDB was positively related to the experience of significant
loss, cognitive confusion, dissatisfaction with life and with
the hospital treatment program, infrequent contact with family
and friends, the absence of religious commitment, and limited
possibilities of discharge.   The degree of observed ISDB was
also associated with negative self-concept and inwardly directed
anger.

4-073 O'Neal, Patricia, Robins, Eli, & Schmidt, Edwin H. (1956).   A
       psychiatric study of attempted suicide in persons over sixty
       years of age.   Archives of Neurology and Psychiatry, 75,
       274-284.

This report was part of a larger study of attempted suicide. In
the paper the authors focused on a study of 109 suicide
attempters, 19 of whom were age 60 and over, and 90 of whom were
under 60. The aim was to describe in detail older attempters
and to compare older to younger attempters. The methods used by
those over 60 were usually violent ones and the most frequently
mentioned precipitating factor was feelings of depression.
Medical problems were also a factor in over half the cases. All
of the older attempters had a clinically diagnosable psychiatric
illness before the attempt.

Comparison of older and younger attempters revealed that older
attempters were more likely to be male (74% vs. 39%), have a
diagnosable psychiatric problem (100% vs. 75%), and less
frequently had problems of love and marriage as well as social
and economic problems.

4-074 Peretti, Peter O., & Wilson, Cedric. (1976).   Anomic and
       egoistic theoretical factors of contemplated suicide among
       voluntary and involuntary retired aged males.   Giornale di
       Gerontologia, 24(2), 119-127. (Abstracts may be found in
       Excerpta Medica, 1977, Sect. 20, 20, No. 1756, p. 314; and
       Excerpta Medica, 1977, Sect. 32, 35, No. 3056, p. 550)

These researchers studied contemplated suicide among voluntarily
and involuntarily retired males.   The aim of the study was to
determine the extent to which Durkheim's concepts of anomic and
egoistic suicide were operating.   It was found that as anomie
and egoism increased so did responses of contemplated suicide
and as the former decreased so did the latter. A tendency
toward increased likelihood of contemplated suicide under both
anomic and egoistic conditions was found for those who were

involuntarily retired.

4-075 Peretti, Peter O., & Wilson, Cedric. (1978-79).   Contemplated
suicide   among   voluntary   and   involuntary   retirees.   Omega:
Journal of Death and Dying, 9, 193-201.

This article begins with a discussion of cultural variations   in
the frequency   and   meaning   of   suicide.   In the United States,
one-fifth of the population is over 45 years of   age,   but   over
three-fifths of   the   suicides in the country come from this age
group. Durkheim's (reference   3-014)   three   types   of   suicide
(anomic,   egoistic,   and   altruistic)   are   discussed and a study
conducted to determine the extent to which anomic   and   egoistic
factors of contemplated suicide might be found among men who had
retired   voluntarily   and   involuntarily.   Men   residing   in   a
Chicago, IL retirement hotel for   the   aged   were   selected   for
interviews (N=140,   mean   age=68.4,   primarily upper-lower class
backgrounds, previously semi-skilled and skilled workers, varied
ethnic backgrounds, good physical and mental health   histories).
The participants were divided into groups according to voluntary
or involuntary   retirement   status as well as their responses to
measures   of   emotional   stability   (anomic   factor)   and
interpersonal   relationships   (egoistic   factor).   Open-ended
questions were   asked   regarding   suicidal   ideation.   The
researchers found   that   men   with   a   high   degree of emotional
stability contemplated   suicide   less   often,   regardless   of
voluntary or   involuntary   retirement   status. Similarly, there
were fewer   contemplated   suicides   among   retirees   who   were
involved in   a   variety   of   interpersonal relationships. After
comparing within groups data, the authors   concluded   that   high
degrees   of   emotional   stability   and   varied   interpersonal
relationships tended to be more important than retirement status
in the contemplation of suicide. Overall, higher anomie led   to
the   greatest   number   of   contemplated   suicides   as Durkheim
predicted. When   comparing   retirement   status,   involuntary
retirees   evidenced   more   anomie   and   egoism than   voluntary
retirees. The hypothesis is made that reducing factors   leading
to anomic   and/or   egoistic   conditions   may reduce contemplated
suicide among retired males.

4-076 Poldinger, Walter J. (1981).   Suicide and attempted   suicide   in
the elderly.   Crisis: International   Journal   of Suicide- and
Crisis-Studies, 2, 117-121.

Using data   from   the   World   Health   Organization,   the   author
presents   a   case   that   the   suicide   rate   for   the   old   is
considerably higher than that for the young.   Suicide   attempts
characterize the   young, whereas completed suicide is more often
the rule for older adults. The author discusses his   own   study
comparing suicide attempts of the young and the old. This study
revealed that   love   and marital problems most often prompted an
attempt in the young. In the   elderly,   loneliness   took   first
place, followed by illness and financial problems. A discussion
of attempted vs. completed suicide then follows in which suicide

is described as a form of auto–aggression and attempted suicide had the function of attracting attention. The elderly are more likely to undertake suicidal behavior from a profound resignation, desperation, and embitterment and therefore with real suicidal intent.

The final section of the paper is devoted to a discussion of suicide prevention. The author argues that to prevent elderly suicide we must be aware of their feelings of loneliness and illness. We need to provide social contact for the old to reduce their social isolation and to provide for their bodily needs as well. Finally, the author recommends that steps be taken to influence the general population to recognize the value of old people and treat them with respect.

4–077   Proudfoot, A. T., & Wright, N. (1972). The physical consequences of self–poisoning by the elderly. Gerontologia Clinica, 14, 24–31.

The authors attempt to investigate the role of the physical consequences of poisoning in the higher mortality rates from suicide in the elderly. Between 1967 and 1969, 160 patients aged 65 and over were admitted to the Regional Poisoning Treatment Centre in Edinburgh (Scotland). Poisonings were classified as intentional or accidental and the intentional poisonings among the elderly were compared with those among younger (under age 65) patients comprising all 1968 admissions. Elderly patients were more likely to use barbiturates and carbon monoxide for intentional self–poisoning. The authors suggested that the elderly are less physically able to cope with drugs with complex actions (i.e., tricyclic antidepressants and non–barbiturate hypnotics). The blood barbiturate levels of the elderly patients were no different than those of the younger patients. The hypothesis that frail, aged patients, with underlying physical illnesses may be more susceptible to large overdoses of barbiturates is presented and rejected. The suggestion is made that elderly patients who self–poison may die from their social isolation or greater efforts to avoid discovery, which prevent them from reaching the intensive medical care they require.

4–078   Quido, M. (1970). Suicide attempts in adolescents and the elderly: A comparative study. In Richard Fox (Ed.), Proceedings: Fifth international conference for suicide prevention, London, September 24–27, 1969 (pp. 37–40). Vienna: International Association for Suicide Prevention.

A study of 131 patients was conducted within a 2 year period, looking at differences in suicidal behavior for the young, middle aged, and old. More frequent suicide attempts were seen in the young (14–25) and the old (55+) than among middle–aged adults. Suicide attempts were far more frequent among girls than boys in adolescence. The most often chosen method was drug overdose for these young people and family integration was weak as was social integration. Attempted suicide was often a result of failed love relationships while psychiatric illness was rare in this group. In the elderly group, equal numbers of men and women attempted suicide. Drug overdose was less often chosen as the method than was seen for the young. Wrist slashing, asphyxiation, and multiple methods were more often used by the elderly. Two-thirds of the elderly attempters had psychiatric troubles formerly, and one-third had experienced some material or emotional problem (such as serious physical illness or loss of a child).

4-079   Rico-Velasco, Jesus, & Mynko, Lizbeth. (1973). Suicide and marital status: A changing relationship? _Journal of Marriage and the Family_, _35_, 239-244.

The authors attempt to demonstrate that marital status per se is not an important factor in determining the suicidal immunity of married persons. A total of 907 cases was reported as suicides by the Department of Health of the city of Columbus and Franklin County, Ohio between 1960 and 1970. Cases with unreported marital status (N=8) and whose ages were below 14 years were excluded from the analyses. The hypotheses were as follows: more males than females kill themselves regardless of marital status; suicide rates are substantially higher among single persons than among the married population; divorced men have a higher rate of suicide than the undivorced; and divorced women have a higher rate of suicide than undivorced women, but lower than for divorced men. These hypotheses were generated from previous research and tested among the Ohio suicidal sample. The first hypothesis was supported. The mean annual suicide rate for males was higher than that for females, regardless of marital status (rates of 21.97 and 8.25 overall for males and females). The second hypothesis was not supported as married persons showed a higher mean annual suicide rate than single persons (14.37 vs. 10.24, respectively). In particular, the annual suicide rate for married females (8.00) was almost double that for single females (4.20). The authors conclude that the myth of suicide as less frequent among the married must be revised. The third hypothesis was tested by including the race and age of subjects. The variability between the mean annual suicide rate diminished when race was controlled. Additionally, the incidence of suicide was found to vary directly with age, the risk increasing as chronological age increased, whether the group was married, single, divorced, widowed, or separated. However, the rates for widowed and divorced men increased as age increased. Race could not be introduced as a controlling factor with age and sex because data for ethnic groups by marital status, sex, and age simultaneously were not reported or available. For females, the age hypothesis was totally confirmed regardless of marital status. The authors again conclude that the marriage hypothesis seems to be rejected. Overall, the relationship between marital status and suicide appears to be changing, especially comparing married to single persons. The hypothesis that married persons have lower mean annual suicide rates than single persons was rejected in this study. The third hypothesis regarding the differential suicide rates between widowed and divorced cannot be rejected, however, the inconsistent results in this sample suggest the need for further study. The authors conclude that our rapidly changing society may be exerting a reversing influence on the relationship between marital status and suicide.

4-080   Reed, Janie, Camus, Joan, & Last, John M. (1985). Suicide in Canada: Birth-cohort analysis. Canadian Journal of Public Health, 76, 43-47.

The authors compared suicide rates for birth cohorts between 1921 and 1980 to determine if the pattern established in Alberta by Solomon and Hellon (1980, reference 4-094) for higher suicide risk with aging occurred nationally. Suicide rates for each birth cohort were gleaned from official government data. Age-specific suicide rates were calculated and rearranged according to birth cohort. Solomon and Hellon's Alberta results were replicated on a national level; that is, suicide rates for each successive birth cohort rose from 1911 to 1961. The birth cohorts exhibited fairly consistent patterns except for a dramatic increase in the 1911 cohort for age groups 20-24 and 24-29. However, these peaks occurred during the period of the Great Depression of the 1930s which have been shown by cross-sectional studies to have a higher suicide rate. Another major difference was found between male and female suicide, with male suicide peaking at about three times that of female suicide. Males also showed a larger increase with successive cohorts while female patterns of suicide had declined with successive cohorts. The authors recommend further study of increases in male suicides.

4-081   Robins, Lee N., West, Patricia A., & Murphy, George E. (1977). The high rate of suicide in older white men: A study testing ten hypotheses. Social Psychiatry, 12, 1-20.

The goal of this study was to investigate the relationship of various beliefs and behaviors to suicidal thoughts and attempts in men. To reach their goal, the authors interviewed a sample of black and white men between the ages of 45 and 65. The sample of 209 men was drawn from three sources: Malcolm Bliss Mental Health Center in St. Louis, City Hospital Medical Clinic, and the Labor Health Institute, a prepaid medical facility run by the Teamster's Union in St. Louis. All subjects were given a structured, personal interview, followed by the Bender-Gestalt Background Interference Procedure to detect brain damage. Hospital records were used to obtain official psychiatric diagnoses. In the interview the subjects were asked questions such as "Has there ever been a time when you thought about taking your own life?" to determine suicidal thoughts or attempts.

There were 10 total hypotheses tested that were drawn from

sociology and psychology. Examples of hypotheses include: social integration protects against suicide; strong religious beliefs protect against suicide; alcoholism is associated with suicide. Results confirmed that suicidal thoughts and behaviors are less frequent in the general sample (Labor Health Institute) than in the psychiatric or medical samples. In the psychiatric and medical samples suicide attempts were much more common among whites than among blacks. Six of the ten hypotheses were supported in whole or in part. Suicidal patients were more socially isolated, more often knew others who had committed suicide, more often felt no pride in aging, more often approved suicide in some circumstances, less often believed in an afterlife, and more often had been depressed and had a family history of depression. Those who had attempted suicide showed no signs of organic brain syndrome. A comparison of black-white differences revealed that certain factors were more prevalent among whites than blacks, perhaps explaining the higher rates of suicide for older white men For example, more whites were unmarried, knew someone who had committed suicide, more often felt no pride in aging, and had a family history of depression.

4-082   Ruzicka, L. T. (1976).   Suicide,   1950–1971.   World Health Statistics Report, 29, 396–413.

Problems with collecting and recording suicide statistics are discussed. Underreporting is the result of administrative and organizations problems, as well as deficiencies of official registration, lack of clear definition, and the tendency to conceal the true facts. The author discusses several problems with comparing suicide statistics from different countries such as differing collection methods and definitions of suicide. In countries where the church is very strong, for example, the tendency may be to search for another label for cause of death. Variation between certifiers of death are large. The author concludes that international comparison of suicide death records and rates should be done carefully with the limitation and differences in mind.

The World Health Organization sent questionnaires to 65 countries to gather data on suicide from 1950 to 1971. Data were available for 54 countries and suicide rates were calculated. In all countries rates were higher for males than for females. In some European countries suicide rates are extremely high (Hungary, Denmark) while in others the rates are very low (Ireland, Italy, Spain). Suicide was found to peak in two life periods: adolescence and old age. Isolation, disease, and bereavement were factors noted to be related to the high rate of suicide in old age. In a few countries a direct increase in suicide with age is not found. In Japan, for example, suicide rates for males have been declining for all ages. The article includes several excellent graphs and tables portraying the fluctuations in suicide rates by age and gender.

4-083   Sainsbury, Peter. (1962a).   Suicide in later life.   Gerontolgia

Clinica, 4, 161-170.

The author utilizes official suicide rates specific for age and sex for several countries to discuss the relation of suicide to mental illness. The relation between depressive symptomatology, physical illness, and suicidal behavior is discussed, as well as the social factors evidenced in old age (loneliness, bereavement, economic deprivation, and retirement). Recommendations are made regarding recognition and intervention in cases of potential suicide, and the need for social legislation to meet the needs of the elderly.

4-084   Sainsbury, Peter. (1962b). Suicide in the middle and later years. In Herman T. Blumenthal (Ed.), Aging around the world: Medical and clinical aspects of aging (pp. 97-105). New York: Columbia University Press.

The author defines the extent of the problem of suicide in middle and late life in England using official statistics. Of the 60 causes of death in middle-aged males, suicide ranked 11th, while in those 65 and above it ranked 19th. Sainsbury also compares the factors in suicide among various age groups based on his earlier research. Interpersonal problems and family quarrels most often preceded suicide in the young and least in the old age group. Physical illness was not a factor in the suicides of young people, however, it was the major factor in late life suicide. Loneliness was another factor in suicide of the old. Finally, the loss of employment was an important factor in the suicides of both the young and middle aged, whereas the lack of employment was more important in elderly suicide.

4-085   Sainsbury, Peter. (1963). Social and epidemiological aspects of suicide with special reference to the aged. In Richard H. Williams, Clark Tibbitts, & Wilma Donahue (Eds.), Processes of aging: Social and psychological perspectives, Volume II (pp. 153-175). New York: Atherton Press.

The author addresses the epidemiology of suicide in the aged, defining the extent of the problem in England and Wales and exploring the causes of the problem, as well as offering methods to guide prevention and treatment. Sainsbury notes that in England and Wales (1949-1953) suicide was the 5th most common cause of death for males 20-34 and the 12th most common cause of death for males 44-64. It was only the 20th leading cause of death for males 65 and above. Suicide increases with age, but it is in fact a more prevalent cause of death in younger ages. Analyzing data from various countries, Sainsbury found that suicide decreased after 65 in the higher social classes and increased in the lower ones. In most European countries the suicide rate was lower in rural areas. In London suicide was positively correlated with social isolation and negatively correlated with high economic status. A significantly higher proportion of the older suicides lived alone. In war time

suicide decreased while in periods of economic depression it
decreased most in younger age groups and least in middle-aged
groups. Physical illness was a factor in suicide of the old but
much less so at younger ages. Similarities and dissimilarities
between depression and suicide were briefly discussed. In terms
of prevention, Sainsbury calls for provision of a satisfactory
social role for the old.

4-086 Sainsbury, Peter. (1968).   Suicide and depression.   In Alec
Coppen & Alexander Walk (Eds.), Recent developments in affective
disorders: A symposium (pp. 1-13).   Kent: Headley Brothers,
Special Publication No. 2, British Journal of Psychiatry.

In this special publication, Sainsbury presents a review of
research findings and official statistics regarding suicide.
Among the statements for which he presents evidence are: one in
ten deaths between the ages of 25 and 34 and one in three deaths
among college students are caused by suicide; perhaps half of
those who commit suicide have depressive illnesses. The author
disagrees with the view that differences in suicide rates
between nations and between districts within a country are due
to methods of reporting suicide. Rather, the differences should
be seen as a social phenomenon. Consequently, the problem is no
longer of defining suicide, but of defining the social
characteristics or personality types associated with suicide.
Based on statistics current when Sainsbury wrote this article,
suicide in women was increasing, largely because the rate for
elderly women had risen significantly. Suicide in men had for
the most part decreased in most countries due to the decline in
younger men.   The author concludes that if suicide is a
barometer of mental well-being, elderly women are apparently
becoming more at risk. Overall, however, women still commit
suicide less than men.

In both sexes, suicide rates nearly always increase sharply with
age. Between the second and third decades the rates doubles,
and in males a peak is usually reached at about 65 but it
usually occurs about 10 years earlier in women. The author
hypothesized that suicide is directly related to social
processes and societal attitudes toward the aged.   Social
factors relate in a predictable way to the incidence of suicide
in a community, although the associations may not be causal.
Durkheim's concept of social isolation is seen as a particularly
useful one in the study of suicide. The practical outcome of
research in social isolation has been to target at-risk groups
in the community as well as to focus efforts of preventive
programming.

Sainsbury focuses on suicide rates in various population groups.
Depression was found to be highly correlated with suicide cases
in Sussex. Overall, one in every six patients diagnosed as
manic-depressive died of suicide, a rate 36 times higher than
that of the general population. Additionally, the risk of
suicide is much higher in elderly depressives.   Other

demographic variables related to suicide risk were sex (higher risk for males), marital status (risk is increased for the divorced or widowed particularly in the early months after widowhood), family history of suicide (higher risk if suicide attempts have been completed by family members), and a past history of personal suicidal attempts. Clinical symptoms which are commonly believed to be associated with suicide are agitation, persistent insomnia, marked feelings of guilt or inadequacy, and delusions of disease. These clinical symptoms associated with depresssion are thought to increase the risk of suicide.

Finally, the relationship between endocrine physiology and suicide is discussed. In particular, the involutional period in women may similarly predispose to depression and suicide. Physical illness is often accompanied by depression and the incidence of physical illness in cases of suicide was higher than in the general population. The characteristics of a depressed person who is a high risk for suicide include: an over 40 male with an endogenous type of depression. One of his parents will have committed suicide during his childhood, and he will have threatened or attempted suicide. His illness will either have been of short duration or he may recently have been released from the hospital; he will be living alone. He will probably complain about feelings of hopelessness and worthlessness and loss of energy rather than his adverse circumstances. He will also probably be drinking heavily. Recommendations for prevention are be aware of the signals of suicidal ideation, question closely person with affective disorders regarding suicidal ideation, in ambiguous cases admission to a hospital for evaluation is recommended, treatment should be thorough with clear plans for follow-up, and more serious consideration needs to be given to improving the general life situation of the older adult if prevention is to be successful.

4-087   Segal, Bernard E. (1969). Suicide and middle age. *Sociological Symposium*, No. 3, 131–141.

This article summarizes information concerning all known suicides occurring between 1955 and 1967 in New Hampshire. Information presented is based on state death certificates and 1960 U.S. Census figures. Data are presented on suicide incidence by sex, age, and marital status. Basic conclusions drawn from these demographic data include: suicide rates among single men are much higher than among married men, except in the youngest age group (14–24); suicide rates among single women are also higher than for the married except in the oldest age group; for men after age 25 and women up to age 65, there is an interaction between age and marital status (low suicide rates occur among younger, married people; high rates among older non-married persons); and high suicide risk categories can be easily identified (married men over 25 and men 65 years of age and older). Basically, New Hampshire's suicide rates for women are consistent with national rates. For men under 25 and over 65, on the other hand, New Hampshire has higher than national suicide rates. Social integration theory is applied in an attempt to explain the variance in suicide rates between the sexes. Socialization and women's greater willingness to ask for help are presented as areas for further study. This author notes that the frequency (i.e., number) of suicides is highest in middle age (34-64) and asserts that involutional depression may occur in middle age and lead to more difficult to detect suicides. This article is not as focused, however, particularly on middle age as the title would imply.

4-088   Seiden, Richard H., & Freitas, Raymond P. (1980). Shifting patterns of deadly violence. Suicide and Life-Threatening Behavior, 10, 194-209.

The authors present official U.S. suicide data to explore the demographic shift in suicides by age during the period 1966-1975. The reduction in suicide at older ages has been reciprocated by an increase in suicide (and homicide) at younger ages (elderly suicide decreased 12%, youthful suicide increased more than 80%). Based on these official data, young white males account for the recent increases in both suicide and homicide, while nonwhite young men continue to have the highest rates of death by homicide. Several "popular" hypotheses are discussed and discarded by the authors as explaining the suicide rate changes (i.e,. changes in casefinding, changes in classification, and changes in the handling of aggression). Joblessness and lifestyle and behavioral changes are presented as the most promising areas for exploration.

4-089   Sendbuehler, J. M., & Goldstein, S. (1977). Attempted suicide among the aged. Journal of the American Geriatrics Society, 25, 244-248. (Reprinted in Margot Tallmer, Daniel J. Cherico, Austin H. Kutscher, David E. Sanders, & Elizabeth R. Prichard (Eds.) (1980), Thanatological aspects of aging: Selected readings (pp. 24-28). Brooklyn, NY: Highly Specialized Promotions.)

This study involved two suicide-attempter populations from two large Canadian cities, Montreal and Ottawa. The Montreal group was observed over a seven year period and comprised part of a series of 222 consecutive suicide attempt patients admitted to a general hospital because they were in danger of dying. The Ottawa group was observed two years later.

Analyses revealed that older individuals are overrepresented in completed suicides and underrepresented in suicide attempts. The older group of attempters had more physical disorders, more psychoses, and more psychopathology than did the younger attempters. One half of the aged suicide attempters had organic brain syndrome. OBS seems to impair successful completion of suicide by interfering with coordination, planning, determination, and awareness of reality. Paradoxically, the

researchers found that suicide attempters had more
psychopathological problems and a higher degree of psychoses
than those who completed suicide.

4-090   Shepherd, D. M., & Barraclough, B. M. (1980). Work and suicide:
An empirical investigation. British Journal of Psychiatry, 136,
469-478.

The authors employ a case study approach to test Emile
Durkheim's (reference 3-014) theory that work is a major source
of social integration, the loss of which encourages suicide.
They investigated the work histories of 75 completed suicides
(40 males and 35 females) and compared them with those of 150
matched controls to test six specific hypotheses derived from
the theory: suicides (1) show more unemployment, (2) are more
likely to be retired, (3) are more likely to have more sick
leave from work, (4) have more frequent job changes, (5) hold
their jobs for shorter times, and (6) show greater social
mobility. Of the total suicides, 24 were above age 65 and the
mean age for males was 52.3 years and 57.5 for females. Data
sources included inquest reports, medical notes, and extended
personal interviews with those closest to the suicide, or in the
case of controls, with the individuals themselves. General
practitioner and hospital records were also used.

Results of the chi-square statistical analyses basically
supported Durkheim's theory and the hypotheses derived from the
theory. Compared with controls, the suicides had a high level
of occupational loss, were unstable in the performance of their
work roles, and had high risk occupations. The most striking
difference was in unemployment. None of the controls was
unemployed on the index day, but nearly one quarter of the
suicides were. The hypothesis about retirement was not
supported, although there was a trend toward earlier retirement
for suicides (but it was not significant). There was also no
difference in the degree of premature retirement, that is, the
age of early retirement. The age at which all work stopped was
significantly younger for suicides than for controls, however.
This age was prior to 60 more often for suicides than controls.
Controls had more gradual retirement while more abrupt and
complete retirement was characteristic of the suicides.

4-091   Shichor, David, & Bergman, Simon. (1979). Patterns of suicide
among the elderly in Israel. Gerontologist, 19, 487-495.

The authors address the rapid processes of industrialization,
urbanization, and immigration occurring in Israel since 1948 and
compare trends in Jewish suicide in Israel to trends in the
United States. Similarities in the patterns were observed with
more completed suicide among males than females and a
preponderance of suicide among the elderly. However, when the
suicide statistics were examined for the country of origin
(Israel-born, American/European immigrants, Asian/African
immigrants) the pattern differed. The high levels of suicide

among the elderly residing in Israel was predominantly among the European/American immigrant group. Etiology and suicide methods were also discussed. The authors suggest suicidal patterns in Israel may reflect differing social status of the elderly in various ethnic groups.

4-092   Simon, Werner, & Lumry, Gayle K. (1970). Suicide of the spouse as a divorce substitute. Diseases of the Nervous System, 31, 608-612.

The focus of this investigation was factors in marital interactions that were significant determinants in suicidal outcome. Patients at the Minneapolis Veteran's Administration Hospital whose spouses committed suicide (N=9) and former patients who had subsequently committed suicide (N=31) were included in the study sample. Demographic data, psychiatric evaluations, diagnosis and hospital treatment were examined as well as exploration of interpersonal dynamics from the point of view of marital conflict and interaction which reflected temporary adaptation or permanent solution to incompatibility (i.e., divorce or suicide). Of these patients, 60% were found to have serious marital discord; 18 patients were separated or divorced and 5 reported divorce threats. Depression, substance abuse, and strong guilt feelings were also prevalent. The dynamics of the marital relationships were discussed in the framework of the concept of divorce substitution.

4-093   Sims, Mary. (1974). Sex and age differences in suicide rates in a Canadian province: With particular reference to suicide by means of poison. Life-Threatening Behavior, 4, 139-159.

The author presents data obtained from the Statistical Division of the Office of the Registrar General, Department of Vital Statistics on the changes in suicide rates by sex and age from 1950 to 1969 in Ontario, Canada. Changes in method by age and sex for this 20 year period were also analyzed. Analyses revealed an increase in suicide for males and females in the later years of life. The largest amount of increase was in the older age groups and among males. Since 1960 there was a marked increase in suicides by poisonings as well as suicides by drugs and/or alcohol overdose. Men are more prone to use alcohol, whereas women use barbiturates and other prescription drugs.

4-094   Solomon, Mark I., & Hellon, Charles P. (1980). Suicide and age in Alberta, Canada, 1951 to 1977: A cohort analysis. Archives of General Psychiatry, 37, 511-513.

A cohort analysis of 4315 suicide deaths registered in Alberta, Canada's vital statistics between 1951 and 1977 was performed. Five-year birth cohorts were identified and followed as they aged through the period of study. A separate analysis was conducted for men and women. Results revealed a higher rate of suicide in the younger age period (14-19) for each successive cohort, and suicide rates increased directly with age, regardless of gender, for each cohort.

4-095 Solomon, Mark I., & Murphy, George E. (1984). Cohort studies of
suicide. In Howard S. Sudak, Amasa B. Ford, & Norman
B. Rushforth (Eds.), Suicide in the young (pp. 1-14). Boston:
John Wright/PGS Inc.

A discussion of the profile method in examining suicide rate in
various age groups of a population is presented. Since
Durkheim's (1897/1951, reference 3-014) time the consistent
finding was for a rarity of completed suicide in younger persons
and a direct positive relationship between suicide and age,
particularly among white males. Profile analysis can be
utilized to construct charts for age-group suicidal tendency
(age-specific rates) or to examine time periods in which changes
in the profiles can be noted. Recently, a shift has occurred in
the age distribution of suicide with rates among adolescents and
young adults approaching those of the more traditionally high
risk older group (see the section on demography in the present
book for a comparison of suicide rates by age groups). The
general conclusions reached using profile analysis are: (1)
traditionally, suicide risk increased directly with age, (2) the
recent rise in adolescent and young adult suicide has decreased
the tendency for suicide to be classified as an older person's
behavior, and (3) this trend (for increased rates among the
young) is general across North America. The cohort method of
analysis is suggested as an alternative to profile analysis.
The cohort method allows one to track a specific birth cohort
through its' lifetime. Reviewing past official records and
applying the cohort method of analysis shows that each
successive birth cohort since 1950 has not only obtained the age
of 14-19 with a higher suicide rate than that of the preceding
five-year cohort, but continues to exhibit a higher suicide rate
than its predecessor in each subsequent five year period.
Although cohort analysis indicates an elevating trend for
younger suicide, caution must be exerted in interpretation since
only a limited number of time periods for tracing cohort rates
of suicide are available.

4-096 Stack, Steven. (1980). The effects of age composition on
suicide in traditional and industrial societies. Journal of
Social Psychology, 111, 143-144.

A multiple regression analysis of the suicide rate (per 100,000
population) was performed on data from industrial and
traditional societies. Data on suicide were obtained from
United Nations sources, and data on proportion of the nation's
population that was over 65 were obtained from the World Bank.
The analysis revealed that the most important variable affecting
the rate of suicide was proportion of the elderly in the
population (beta=.487, p<.005), followed by the rate of economic
growth (beta=.215, p<.05). The results support the hypothesis
of a direct relationship between suicide and aging, even in a
sample of both industrial and traditional societies.

4-097 Stack, Steven. (1982a). Aging and suicide: A cross-national study. International Journal of Contemporary Sociology, 19, 124-138.

The author tested three major sociological theories of suicide (social integration, anomie, and urbanization) using official suicide statistics collected by the United Nations. The comparative study involved 45 nations from which the proportion of aged in the population was the indicator of social integration. The higher the proportion of aged, the lower the social integration. Rate of economic growth was the indicator of anomie and rapid economic growth indicated higher anomie. Results of the multiple regression analysis revealed that all three independent variables contributed to the variance in the suicide rate of the old. Proportion of the aged in the population, the indicator of social integration, explained the largest portion of variance. The corrected coefficient of determination indicates that 34% of the variation in suicide rate was explained by the three variables. Stack concluded that "nations marked by a high proportion of aged, high rate of economic growth, and relatively large urban population will have relatively high suicide rates."

4-098 Stack, Steven. (1982b). Suicide in Detroit 1975: Changes and continuities. Suicide and Life-Threatening Behavior, 12, 67-83.

Problems (the use of highly aggregated data, the use of non-aggregated data but using summary tables for entire nations, and the overall age, i.e., dated nature, of the research) in the literature on suicide are discussed and a study correcting for these problems is presented. The data for the study are from all persons who died in 1975 in Detroit whose death certificate indicated the cause as suicide (N=193). Data were taken from the death certificates and were therefore limited to marital status, sex, race, age, occupation, industry of employment, place of birth, and the month of suicide. The study was designed to test four broad theories of suicide regarding social integration, economic theory with respect to occupational status, differential socialization theory with respect to sex and race differences, and climatic theory with respect to seasonal variations of suicide. A decline in the incidence of suicide among the divorced was interpreted as due to the decrease in stigma associated with a divorce. Data on suicide rates by age also indicated changes. Younger persons had the highest rate of suicide. The "baby boomers" (24-34 years of age) had the highest overall rate compared to traditional findings of the elderly as highest risk. Stack found evidence that laborers were more than six times more likely to kill themselves than were either professional or technical or managerial workers. This seems to support earlier studies (e.g., Ronald W. Maris, 1969, Social Forces in Urban Suicide, Homewood, IL: Dorsey Press) in which lower rates of suicide were seen in higher social classes. Stack hypothesizes that as unemployment continues to rise, suicide in lower prestige groups will be disproportionately high. These results in Detroit found whites to be twice as likely as blacks to kill themselves. The failure of the race difference in suicide to diminish is attributed to the lack of appreciable advances in the area of residential desegregation (i.e., residential segregation may indicate that blacks have been able to maintain a significantly different culture than whites with respect to norms attached to aggression).   In addition to the race differential, the differences between the sexes were also seen to be constant, with men three times more likely to commit suicide. Stack hypothesizes that women's greater participation in the work force has not adversely affected their suicide rates. When considering age, sex, and race simultaneously, these data show suicide rates to be highest for both black and white males at young ages. Stack declares the existence of a youth suicide epidemic. Finally, the study indicated a large percentage (60%) of the suicides in the spring and fall among the Detroit residents. These peaks are interpreted to mean that the changes in the seasons affect the suicide rates and that fall is the sign of a cold winter which may promote suicidal ideation in an already depressed person.

Stack comments on the need for further study of subpopulations, particularly with the finding of a youth epidemic which is contrary to other literature indicating disproportionate rates of suicide among the elderly. Reformulations in theories explaining why the elderly have high suicide rates, and particularly with respect to age status in social integration theory are recommended.

4-099 Tuckman, Jacob, Youngman, William F., & Bleiberg, Beulah M. (1962). Attempted suicide by adults. Public Health Reports, 77, 604-614.

The authors examine 1112 consecutive attempted suicides by persons 18 years of age and over from 1959-1961 who came to the attention of police in Philadephia, PA. Race, sex, and age distribution figures are reported (males=355, females=757, white=777, nonwhite=335, median age=33). Suicide attempts clearly declined with age for women, whites, and nonwhites; men showed no specific declines with age. These results contrast with those for completed suicide where an increase with age is noted. The authors conclude that attempted suicide is a function of youth, while completed suicide is function of age. Nonwhites were overrepresented in attempted suicide, while women over 45 exhibited suicide attempt rates roughly equivalent to male suicide rates. Of the attempted suicides, 63% used poisons, while other methods included gas or carbon monoxide (12%), cutting or piercing (17%), jumping, hanging, firearms, and drowning (<5%), and combinations of methods (4%). Women used poisons more often than men and men used cutting and piercing more often than women. Whites employed sedatives and tranquilizers more frequently than nonwhites although nonwhites utilized external medicines more often than whites. Most attempts took place in the person's home and the most common motivation was interpersonal difficulty. Recommendations for suicide prevention programs are given, including evaluation and referral services, consultation services for social service and medical providers, community education, development of follow-up procedures, and case finding that results in the identification of salient factors in suicidal behavior.

4-100   Walsh, Dermot, & McCarthy, P. Desmond. (1965). Suicide in Dublin's elderly. Acta Psychiatrica Scandinavica, 41, 227-235.

The official suicide rate in Ireland is the lowest in Europe and one of the lowest in the world. The suggestion has been made that the suicide verdict is avoided due to the influence of Roman Catholicism and the subsequent connotations of a suicide verdict. A survey of suicide over age 60 (N=90) in Dublin was presented to determine if Ireland's official rate was indeed underreported. Following examination of coroners' records, the author concluded that, if Dublin is representative, Ireland does possess one of the lowest European suicide rates.

4-101   Wen, Chi-Pang. (1974). Secular suicidal trend in postwar Japan and Taiwan: An examination of hypotheses. International Journal of Social Psychiatry, 20, 8-17.

This study was conducted in an attempt to broaden knowledge of suicide through description of some unusual trends in Japan and Taiwan. After World War II, Japan and Taiwan, in comparison to other countries, had very high rates of suicide for all age groups. Furthermore, both countries exhibited unique bimodal age distributions for suicide rates. That is, suicide peaks were for ages 14-24 and 45-54+ years of age. By 1964 in Japan and 1970 in Taiwan, the bimodality virtually disappeared with suicide rates similar to those traditionally seen in the United States (i.e., increases with age, with a single peak in old age). One aspect of youth suicide in Japan and Taiwan that is discussed is the methods of suicide. Drug overdoses and chemical poisons are the major means of suicide in the young and the availability of hypnotics and tranquilizers is discussed.

The elderly in Japan and Taiwan also exhibit high suicide rates; from 2 to 6 times higher than among the elderly in the United States. The author discusses the increasing migration of the younger generation to seek employment as well as the expectation on the part of the elderly that they will be cared for by their children. Possibly the unrealisticness of this expectation leads to the increased rate of elderly suicide in Japanese and Taiwanese societies. Elderly persons primarily use hanging or strangulation or poisons in their suicides. Several arguments are presented to refute the stereotype of honor in suicide among Japanese elderly. The rising incidence of youthful suicide, different methods of suicide between the young and the elderly, and the dramatic decrease in suicide in the past decade are primary arguments against the myth of honorable suicide.

Female suicide is also higher in Japan and Taiwan than in the United States. Women in Japan and Taiwan are forced to deal with social intolerance toward divorce, bleak prospects for remarriage, lack of sexual freedom, and the culturally male-dominant chauvinistic attitudes. It is possible that these attitudes affect the female suicide rates.

4-102   Wenz, Friedrich V. (1976). Suicide and marital status: A case of high suicide rate among the widowed. Crisis Intervention, 7(4), 149-161.

4-103   Wenz, Friedrich V. (1977). Marital status, anomie, and forms of social isolation: A case of high suicide rate among the widowed in an urban sub-area. Diseases of the Nervous System, 38, 891-895.

Wenz presents the same findings in both 4-102 and 4-103 above. The study examines the high suicide rates among the widowed in one census tract in Flint, MI and identifies the major social and psychological factors responsible for the unusally high rates among this group. The number of official suicides in the city consisted on 270 cases for the period 1971-1973 and 20 (7.4%; rate=126 per 100,000) cases occurred in the census tract under consideration. Among the cases in this census tract 65% were widowed. A probability area sample was drawn from that tract and 85 interviews were conducted. Information was collected on age, sex, race, etc., and a number of social-psychological scales were administered (Srole's Anomie Scale, Social Isolation in the Present Scale, and Anticipation of Social Isolation in the Future Scale).

An in-depth analysis revealed that the census tract differed in several ways from the city of Flint as a whole. It possessed a greater proportion of nonwhites, foreign-born, and less educated, and a lower proportion of white collar workers, greater residential mobility and proportion of renters, fewer elderly, and a much higher percentage of women in the labor force. Analysis of suicide rates showed that the rate for widowed individuals in this census tract was 11 times greater than for the widowed in Flint. The census tract also had a higher suicide rate for the 45 and older age group than did the remainder of the city. In order to understand the higher rates for widowed persons in this area, the author analyzed data obtained from the sample of 85. Analyses indicated that in this area the widowed are more anomic and see themselves as more socially isolated at present and in the future than do those who are married, single, or divorced. Wenz concludes that as the proportion of widowed increases beyond a certain level in the community, the support system becomes overloaded, resulting in a higher suicide rate. Recommendations are made to focus suicide prevention programs on the widowed at all ages, and to utilize paraprofessional as well as professional helpers in an attempt to reduce social isolation and anomie among the widowed.

4-104   Wenz, Friedrich V. (1979).   Family   constellation   factors,
        depression, and   parent suicide potential. American Journal of
        Orthopsychiatry, 49, 164-167.

        Minimal research has been directed toward assessing the impact
        of the number of children in the family unit on parental
        suicidal thoughts, threats, and   acts.   Although   Durkheim
        (1897/1951, reference 3-014) and Halbwachs (1930/1975, The
        Causes of Suicide, New York: Arno Press) believed children had
        a "protective" effect on the married, more recent research has
        failed to support this hypothesis.   Wenz tests   Durkheim's
        proposition   that   marital   partners   (especially women) are
        protected against suicide risk in direct proportion to the
        number of children they have.   A total of 245 families (243
        parents, 392 children) in which a parent either thought of or
        threatened suicide, and suffered actual self-inflicted damage
        composed the sample. A family was defined as a unit of at least
        one parent and one child under 18 years of age. The number of
        children in the household at the time of the suicide attempt
        (family size) and the ratio of children to adults living in the
        household (family density) were related to the lethality rating
        for both male and female parents, however, family size was the
        strongest predictor variable. There was a tendency for women to
        be "protected" from suicide more by family size. Wenz cites
        studies on psychological well-being which indicate that women
        are more psychologically disturbed than men, and find their
        societal roles more constricting and frustrating, as explanatory
        evidence of the greater importance of family size for women.
        Additional research on family constellation and parent suicide
        is recommended, in particular with regard to step-relationships.
        Because of sample selection criteria, elderly parents were not
        included.   It is the opinion of the present authors that similar
        research which attempts to determine the "protective" effect
        that adult children have for their elderly parents is also
        needed, especially with regard to the number of children, number
        and frequency of visits, geographic proximity, etc.

4-105   Wenz, Friedrich V. (1980). Aging and suicide: Maturation or
        cohort   effect?   International Journal of Aging and Human
        Development, 11, 297-305.

        A survey questionnaire was administered to 314 person within
        four census tracts in Flint, MI. Four questions which could be
        used to develop a Suicide Potential Scale were part of the
        larger questionnaire.   Wenz's results support a cohort model to
        explain suicide.   That is, individuals   establish   suicidal
        patterns at an early age and are more likely to commit suicide
        as they become older. That is, predispositional factors exist
        which determine suicide potential.   It is concluded that
        individuals are more likely to adopt suicidal patterns early in
        life and are thus more likely to complete the suicidal act as
        they become older.

4-106   Whitlock, F. A. (1978).   Suicide,   cancer,   and   depression.

British Journal of Psychiatry, 132, 269–274.

The relationship between depression and malignant diseases is discussed and a review of 1965 to 1967 post–mortem records in Brisbane was completed to identify all cases of suicide aged 50 and above. An additional 50 suicides, in the same age group, from the Brisbane Suicide Study (unpublished results at that time) were added to the sample. Suicides under 50 years of age were deleted from the study due to the relative infrequency of carcinoma deaths in younger persons. A sample of individuals dying from violent deaths, matched for age and sex, was also compiled from post–mortem records to serve as a control group. A total of 273 suicides age 50 and over was recorded. A much higher than expected incidence of neoplasms was found among the suicide victims than among the matched control group ($p<.001$). Seven of the malignant cases in the suicide groups and one malignant case in the control group had not been diagnosed before death (tumors were discovered upon autopsy). Additionally, the extent to which other suicides were informed as to their illness was unknown. Several studies describing depression as a precursor to manifestation of a malignant disease are discussed, as well as the hypotheses that depression may weaken the bodily defenses against circulating neoplastic cells.

4–107   Wilbanks, William. (1982). Trends in violent death among the elderly. International Journal of Aging and Human Development, 14, 167–175.

Although recent media reports indicate an increase in violent crime against the elderly, no data have been provided to support this claim. Wilbank attempts to fill this gap by presenting official data for the aged population. He reports that the elderly are much less likely to die by homicide (or suicide or accident) than other age groups, perhaps due to the greater tendency of the elderly to die from natural causes. [Note: Wilbanks refers to the absolute number of deaths rather than the rates in this statement. See the demographic presentation in Chapter 1 of the present book.] In fact, for the population as a whole the trend is for a decrease from 1960–1975 in violent or accidental death. The only exception to this trend, is for an increase in the homicide rate for the elderly. However, Wilbanks points out that the increase in homicide rates among the aged is accompanied by a decrease in accidental and suicide death, and thus an overall decrease in the total rate of violent death among the elderly. The author encourages additional research exploring specific decreases in accidental and suicidal deaths among the elderly.

4–108   Wold, Carl I. (1971). Sub–groupings of suicidal people. Omega: Journal of Death and Dying, 2, 19–29.

The author reports subgroups of suicidal persons seen at the Los Angeles Suicide Prevention Center in the hope of increasing the

accuracy of suicide prediction and the development of new
treatment methods based on the identified characteristics and
needs of varying subgroups. The subgroups were determined by
three methods: clinical, clustering, and factor analytic
techniques. Records of 500 randomly selected clients were
utilized. The clinical subgroups were composed of the following
thematic areas: discarded women, violent men, middle-age
depression, harlequin, I can't live without you, I can't live
with you, adolescent-family crisis, down and out, old and alone,
and chaotic. The old and alone group was 60+, often suffered
from a debilitating illness, was lonely and depressed, had
outlived most of their friends and relatives, and saw life as a
major effort. They were not chaotic or impulsively suicidal.
The clinical subgroupings were then subjected to cluster
analysis. Age, sex, and acute versus chronic suicide problems
emerged as three dimensions. Each dimension is discussed in
terms of characteristics of the group, and recommended
treatment. The author cautions the reader to interpret the
results as tentative until complete analysis is conducted.

4-109 Wolff, Kurt. (1969). Depression and suicide in the geriatric
patient. Journal of the American Geriatrics Society, 17,
668-672.

4-110 Wolff, Kurt. (1970a). The emotional rehabilitation of the
geriatric patient (pp. 97-103, "Depression and suicide in the
geriatric patient"). Springfield, IL: Thomas.

4-111 Wolff, Kurt. (1970b). Observations on depression and suicide in
the geriatric patient. In Kurt Wolff (Ed.), Patterns of
self-destruction: Depression and suicide (pp. 33-42).
Springfield, IL: Thomas.

4-112 Wolff, Kurt. (1971, July). The treatment of the depressed and
suicidal geriatric patient. Geriatrics, 26, 64-69.

Wolff presents the same study results in each of the above four
references, 4-109, 4-110, 4-111, and 4-112. A study was made of
the longitudinal case histories of 200 elderly male veterans
(mean age=64) who had been in the Coatesville Veterans
Administration Hospital for at least two years. Patients were
classified into two groups: (A) those with a history of
depression and no suicidal episodes, and (B) those with a
history of depression and past suicidal ideation. Through
careful review of cases and in-depth interviews with families,
data were gathered on diagnosis, psychodynamics, prognosis, and
treatment methods.

Patients in Group A differed markedly from those in Group B. In
Group A symptoms of depression were related to "loss" (physical,
health, independence, or social status) or failure. In Group B
symptoms of depression were related to compulsivity. These
patients were ambitious, hard workers, relatively rigid, and
inflexible in their behaviors. The patients in Group A were of

the passive-dependent type while those of Group B had a psychotic depressive reaction.

The author points out that treatment programs for the two types of patients must take into account these differences. He recommends supportive individual or group psychotherapy for members of Group A to help them deal with their loss and feelings of failure. For members of Group B, on the other hand, he recommends electro-convulsive therapy. In both groups anti-depressant drugs can be effective.

4-113 Yap, P. M. (1963). Aging and mental health in Hong Kong. In Richard H. Williams, Clark Tibbitts, & Wilma Donahue (Eds.), Processes of aging: Social and psychological perspectives, Volume II (pp. 176-191). New York: Atherton Press.

The author focuses on rates of psychiatric referral and attempted and completed suicide in Hong Kong from 1956-1958. Failing a census survey, the number of cases of combined inpatients and outpatients referred for treatment for the first time provides the most accurate indication of the extent of mental disease in a community. Calculating these rates revealed the rate is higher for elderly females than for elderly males in Hong Kong and the rate is considerably lower in Hong Kong than in Western countries in the same time period. Thus, the rate of mental illness overall is considerably lower in aged Chinese than in aged Westerners. Yap also found that the rate declined with age.

A study of suicide rates in Hong Kong revealed less mental health and happiness among the aged. Examining suicide and attempted suicide curves by age and sex, based on a total of 263 and 894 cases, respectively, Yap found that the male suicide curve rises with age and the female curve starts to rise rapidly after age 55 and overtakes the male curve. To explain the vulnerability of aged women in Hong Kong, Yap takes an historical perspective. He points out that in the patriarchal society of Peking 43 years ago, the suicide rate for aged females was much lower than in the industrializing, modernizing Hong Kong of the 1960s. The old culture gave more prestige and support to older women. The fast paced economic and social changes recently experienced in Hong Kong have left aged women, many of whom are illiterate, poor, and widowed, in a more vulnerable position.

5
NON-ENGLISH LANGUAGE WORKS

The references in this chapter are considerations of elderly suicide written in languages other than English. A total of 12 different languages are represented. The annotations that accompany some of the references are taken either from reading the original articles, or in most cases, from an English abstract that summarized the article contents. When abstracts were annotated rather than the entire article, the abstract may have occurred either as part of the original article (Note: those articles for which an abstract appears in the journal in English are noted in parentheses with the notation "English abstract") or appeared in one of the several abstract sources that are noted for many of the articles. In cases where the annotation appearing here is a synopsis of an abstract of the original article, only a brief summary is possible. This is necessary because of the limited information generally available in abstracts regarding methodology, results, and discussion of the implications of the results. Below, the sources of English abstracts (when available) and the abbreviations used for those sources appear in parentheses following the full references citation (see the Introduction for more information on abstract sources):

> Abstracts in Criminology and Penology [ACP] now called
>   Criminology and Penology Abstracts [CPA]
> Excerpta Medica [EM]
> Psychological Abstracts [PA]
> Sociological Abstracts [SA]

5–001   Anger, H. (1977, February). [Social psychological aspects of suicide in old age]. Aktuelle Gerontologie, 7(2), 75–80. /*GERMAN*/ (English abstract) (Abstracts: EM, 1978, Sect. 20, 21, No. 1079, p. 200; EM, 1977, Sect. 32, 37, No. 2259, p. 411)

5–002   Aubry, H. (1974). [Incidence of late suicide among former psychiatric patients]. Schweizer Archiv fur Neurologie, Neurochirurgie und Psychiatrie, 114(2), 303–337. /*FRENCH*/ (English abstract) (Abstracts: ACP, 1975, 15, No. 702, p. 187; PA, 1975, 54, No. 9916, p. 1233; EM, 1975, Sect. 32, 31, No. 1433, p. 249)

This study investigated the suicide rate among 5661 former hospitalized psychiatric patients born between 1873 and 1897. These rates were compared to that for the same age groups in the general population of Switzerland. The results indicated that (1) between 1942 and 1962 a total of 1891 of the patients died with 107 of the deaths by suicide, (2) the suicide level for the psychiatric patients was 5.6% compared to 1.76% and .66% in men and women in the population in general, respectively, (3) the differences between the sexes for suicide were less pronounced in the psychiatric patient group, (4) by diagnosis, the highest levels of suicide were seen for manic and manic-depressive patients (11% for men and 10% for women), followed in order by alcoholics (7.3% for men, 5.4% for women), and then psychogenic and psychopathic disorders (6.8% for men, 5.4% for women). Limitations of the data are discussed.

5-003   Bocker, F. (1975, February 7). [Suicide in the elderly]. Munchener Medizinische Wochenschrift, 117(6), 201-204. /*GERMAN*/ (English abstract) (Abstracts: EM, 1976, Sect. 20, 19, No. 294, p. 53; EM, 1976, Sect. 32, 33, No. 1283, p. 224)

This article reviews the literature on elderly suicide and presents data on German suicides by age, sex, and psychiatric diagnosis. The author suggests that loneliness, isolation, and physical illness are factors in elderly suicide and urges doctors to prevent suicide among their aged patients.

5-004   Bohm, M., Conradi, M., & Rissmann, W. (1983). [Suicidal acts in advanced age - Some characteristics and rehabilitative approaches.] Zeitschrift fur Alternforschung, 38, 51-55. /*GERMAN*/ (English abstract)

5-005   Bojanovsky, J. (1975). [Suicide in the divorced and widowed]. Fortschritte der Medizin, 93(14), 714-717. (Abstract: EM, 1976, Sect. 32, 33, No. 442, p. 76)

5-006   Bojanovsky, J., & Bojanovsky, A. (1976, May). [The suicidal risk period after partner loss through divorce or death: An epidemiological study]. Nervenarzt, 47(5), 307-309. (Abstract: EM, 1977, Sect. 20, 20, No. 1780, p. 318; EM, 1977, Sect. 32, 35, No. 3054, p. 550)

5-007   Bungard, W. (1977, February). [Isolation, loneliness and suicidal ideas in the aged]. Aktuelle Gerontologie, 7(2), 81-89. /*GERMAN*/ (English abstract) (Abstracts: EM, 1977, Sect. 20, 20, No. 3471, p. 630; EM, 1977, Sect. 32, 36, No. 3785, p. 701)

Suicidal ideation among a group of 406 respondents above the age of 65 was studied. Suicidal ideation was found to be the result of both a loss of or social denial of intimate and personally important relationships. Suicidal ideas were also related to feelings of loneliness but the latter was unrelated to the quantity of social contacts. The results further indicated the importance of the voluntariness of the disengagement as well as the constancy of the life style.

5-008 Cahn, L. A. (1965). [Suicide and attempted suicide in old age]. Tijdschrift voor Sociale Geneeskunde, 43(25), 898-903. /*GERMAN*/

5-009 Cahn, L. A. (1968, July 1). [Depressive states in the elderly]. Tijdschrift voor Ziekenverpleging, 21, 529-534. /*DUTCH*/

5-010 Chatagnon, P., Chatagnon, C., & Wilkin, M.-O. (1960). [A case of enforced retirement: Autothanasia; assistance of elderly people]. Annales Medico-Psychologiques, 118(5), 891-905. /*FRENCH*/

5-011 Chikazawa, K. (1974, January). [Statistical observation of suicide by the aged: Its relationship with the welfare problem]. Japanese Journal of Nursing Art, 20, 54-63. /*JAPANESE*/

5-012 Ciompi, L. (1966, April). [Suicide and suicide attempts in old age]. Revue Medicale de la Suisse Romande, 86(4), 260-262. /*FRENCH*/

5-013 Courbon, P., & Rousset, S. (1936). [Impulsions to suicide in an old epileptic patient]. Annales Medico-Psychologiques, 94, 765-770.

5-014 Danneel, R. (1975, December 23). [Seasonal differences in the frequency of suicide in youth and old age]. Archiv fur Psychiatrie und Nervenkrankheiten, 221(1), 11-13. /*GERMAN*/ (English abstract) (Abstracts: PA, 1976, 56, No. 10090, p. 1208; EM, 1976, Sect. 20, 19, No. 3385, p. 598; EM, 1976, Sect. 32, 34, No. 2644, p. 476)

A study of 1704 suicides is presented which are comprised of 852 younger suicides (born 1940-1961) and 852 older suicides (born 1878-1904). Danneel found that suicides vary over the year for both the young and old in Germany and varies differentially for the two age groups. More specifically, for the young suicides are highest in autumn and winter while for the old the peak times are spring and summer. These differences were statistically significant.

5-015 De Alarcon, R. (1968, September). [Earlier diagnosis of depressions of the aged]. Revista de Medicina de la Universidad de Navarra, 12(3), 193-207. /*SPANISH*/ (Abstract: PA, 1971, 45, No. 4527, p. 482)

This investigation studied the presence of hypochondriacal symptoms in 73 male and 79 female individuals over the age of 60 who had been treated for depression at a geriatric psychiatric hospital. Among these subjects, 63.81% displayed hypochondriacal symptoms at some stage of their depression. In 45 of the subjects these symptoms were manifested from 2 weeks to 9 months before the appearance of depressive symptoms. All subjects with the hypochondriacal symptoms had visited a physician and/or general hospitals but had not been psychiatrically examined. Only after either great agitation or a suicide attempt was the proper diagnosis of depression made. Nearly 25% of the patients with hypochondriacal symptoms attempted suicide compared to only 3% of those without such symptoms. The diagnostic utility of hypochondriacal symptoms for early diagnosis of depression is suggested and a simple method for physicians to help in excluding the possibility of depression is presented.

5-016   De las Matas Davila, J. S. (1976, November). [Discussions on old age and suicide]. Folia Clinica Internacional, 26(11), 512-526. /*SPANISH*/

The author discusses several changes related to aging which could be factors in their high suicide rate. Biological and psychological changes, particularly confusion and memory loss, are noted. Negative attitudes toward the old and increased social isolation among the aged are also cited as contributory factors.

5-017   Decke, D. (1975, September). [Dispensary care of suicidal cases in later life]. Psychiatrie, Neurologie und Medizinische Psychologie, 27(9), 534-541. /*GERMAN*/ (English abstract)

5-018   Descloux, A. (1971). [Depression and suicide]. Zeitschrift fur Praventivmedizin, 16(1), 97-103. /*FRENCH*/ (Abstract: EM, 1972, Sect. 20, 15, No. 1566, p. 255)

5-019   Drdkova, S., & Zemek, P. (1976, February). [Development of the suicide rate in people above 65 years in Czechoslovakia in 1919-1971]. Sbornik Lekarsky, 78(2), 45-52. /*CZECH*/

5-020   Elozo, E. P. (1973). [Suicidal tendencies in depressive psychoses of old age]. Zhurnal Nevropatologii i Psikhiatrii imeni S. S. Korsakova, 73(3), 431-434. /*RUSSIAN*/ (English abstract) (Abstracts: EM, 1974, Sect. 32, 29, No. 711, p. 123; EM, 1974, Sect. 20, 17, No. 713, p. 118)

A study of 226 suicidal psychotic patients found that 23.45% had attempted suicide while the remainder had thoughts and wishes. For these 226 patients, their psychoses had begun after age 40 and their suicidal tendencies were associated with depression. Males were most likely to be the attempters while females expressed ideation verbally. Relationships (undesignated in the abstract) were established between the frequency of the suicidal thoughts, the type and form of the disorder.

5-021   Elwitz, J. (1980). [The importance of disease in suicide among old people] (Doctoral dissertation, Universitat zu

Erlangen-Nurnberg,   1977).   <u>Dissertation   Abstracts International-C: European abstracts</u>, <u>40</u>, No. 4/3794c, 470C.

The only conditions which the author found to motivate suicide attempts other than severe endogenous depression were organic diseases with great pain (e.g., carcinoma at late stages, degenerative motor apparatus diseases in advanced stages, and angina pectoris). The diseases were especially important in the attempt if they were seen as only part of the motivational picture. The author notes the generally high resistance to suicide among the old with physical problems and suggests that suicide only becomes a thought when social relationships and feelings of social identity are weakened or lost.

5-022   Fedotov, D. C., & Chudin, A. S. (1976).   [Suicide attempts in the involutional and aged periods]. <u>Zhurnal Nevropatologii i Psikhiatrii imeni S. S. Korsakova</u>, <u>76</u>(3), 405-409.   /*RUSSIAN*/ (English   abstract) (Abstracts: <u>EM</u>, 1976,   Sect. 20,   <u>19</u>, No. 3843, p. 676;   <u>EM</u>,   1976,   Sect. 32,   <u>34</u>,   No. 3422, pp. 613-614)

Based on their study of 76 patients over age 50 (range=51 to 87) who attempted suicide, the authors identified the main syndromes during which suicide was attempted.   Of these 76, were 15 alcoholics (13 males, 2 females).   The other syndromes identified were anxious-depressive, depressive-hypochondriasis, and depressive-delusional.   The authors also discussed the following factors which contributed to suicidal tendency: involutional changes, somatic disorders, and psychogenic traumas. They found that following the suicidal act patients suffered from various mental disturbances that required psychiatric treatment.

5-023   Feuerlein, W. (1977, February).   [Causes,   motivations   and tendencies of suicidal acts in old age]. <u>Aktuelle Gerontologie</u>, <u>7</u>(2), 67-74. /*GERMAN*/ (English abstract) (Abstracts: <u>EM</u>, 1977, Sect. 20, <u>20</u>, No. 3470, p. 630; <u>EM</u>, 1977,   Sect. 32,   <u>36</u>, No. 3784, p. 701)

A total of 125 patients over the age of 65 who were suicidal were compared to a control group of 3004 suicidal patients below the age of 65.   The major psychiatric diagnosis was depression (50% of old group and 33% of control group).   Among the motivations for suicide were conflicts with spouses or other relatives (24%), fear of somatic illness, and social isolation in that order of frequency of mention. Occupational and economic problems were mentioned by <u>none</u> of the elderly attempters. One of the factors promoting lessened suicide prevention that is mentioned is modifying attitudes toward the old.

5-024   Gelpi, I. L., & Papeschi, A. J. (1960).   [Mental hygiene in geriatrics: Suicides and accidents in old age]. <u>Semana Medica</u>, <u>116</u>(39), 1307-1312. /*SPANISH*/

The main objective of this article is to examine mental health problems of the old. The authors note that compared to other age groups the old suffer from a large number of mental health problems and from more serious problems. In their discussion of suicide as a major problem of the old the authors focus on three factors: living environment, family relationships, and work conditions. The old are more often retired and living alone, cut off from relations with their family. Another factor noted in connection with suicide is the biological changes which accompany aging. The authors conclude that since the elderly are the most at risk for suicide, more attention should be paid to this group and more education of health professionals working with the old is needed.

5-025 Graux, P. (1974, August-September). [Suicide of the aged]. Lille Medical, 19(7), 754-755. /*FRENCH*/ (Abstract: EM, 1975, Sect. 20, 18, No. 2229, p. 382)

5-026 Groschke-Bachmann, D. (1982). [Suicide in old age: A sociological view.] Aktuelle Gerontologie, 12(2), 60-63. /*GERMAN*/ (English abstract)

5-027 Gruhle, H. W. (1941). [Suicide and old age]. Zeitschrift fur Altersforschung, 3, 21. /*GERMAN*/

5-028 Gruneberg, F. (1977, February). [Phenomenlology of suicidal actions in old age]. Aktuelle Gerontologie, 7(2), 91-100. /*GERMAN*/ (English abstract) (Abstracts: EM, 1977, Sect. 32, 37, No. 352, p. 67; EM, 1978, Sect. 20, 21, No. 337, p. 63)

5-029 Gyorgy, G. (1977, May 29). [Relationship between age and selection of suicide form]. Orvosi Hetilap, 118(22), 1283-1284. /*HUNGARIAN*/

5-030 Hedri, A. (1967). [Suicide in advanced age]. Schweizer Archiv fur Neurologie, Neurochirurgie und Psychiatrie, 100(1), 179-202. /*GERMAN*/

5-031 Hedri, A. (1969, October). [Suicide in old age as a problem of preventive medicine]. Therpeutische Umschau, Revue Therpeutique, 26(10), 571-573. /*GERMAN*/ (Abstract: EM, 1970, Sect. 20, 13, No. 1681, p. 275)

5-032 Hedri, A. (1978, October). [Stress of the elderly]. Aktuelle Gerontologie, 8(10), 537-538. /*GERMAN*/ (English abstract)

5-033 Hoshi, M. (1977, October). [Activities of a home helper. Psychological processes of the aged; an observation of a case resulting in suicide]. Kangogaku Zasshi, 41(10), 1070-1072. /*JAPANESE*/

5-034 Jenson, K. (1979, December 12). [Acute poisoning: Poisoning in adults mostly blamed on suicide]. Sygeplejersken, Dansk

Sygeplejerad, 79(49), 18–21. /*DANISH*/

5–035 Knipscheer, C. P. (1977, March). [The suicide rate for older people: A demographic and sociologic reanalysis]. Nederlands Tijdschrift voor Gerontologie, 8(1), 20–24. /*DUTCH*/ (English summary) (Abstracts: EM, 1977, Sect. 32, 37, No. 2638, p. 480; PA, 1978, 60, No. 3274, p. 368)

Kruijt (e.g., 1977, reference 4–042) and others noted the decline in the suicide rate for the old since World War II in several European countries. In this analysis of Netherlands' data, Knipscheer found that the declines were highly correlated with the decreasing proportion of widowed individuals over the age of 60, especially for males. This change in marital status proportions should be taken into account in explanations of elderly suicide trends. Comparable data analyses in other countries to determine the effect of this phenomenon more generally are also needed.

5–036 Kockott, G. (1981).   [Attempted suicide in old age.] Fortschritte der Medizin, 99(26), 1049–1056.   /*GERMAN*/ (English abstract)

This study compared three age groups of patients who had attempted suicide: under 40 years, 40–64, and older than 64 years. A comparison with distributions of characteristics in the general ("normal") population is also made. Men were underrepresented in the two younger age groups but not in old age. The same was found among male foreigners. Divorced individuals were overrepresented in all age groups while single persons were overrepresented in the two young groups. In all age groups the ratio of married patients was underrepresented while the widowed were equally represented in all attempters groups compared with the ratio in the normal population. Diagnoses of depression increased with age while others decreased. The present old attempters displayed similar motives for their attempts to those seen in another study of much younger attempters but displayed different motives than seen among elderly completers. It is concluded therefore that older attempters and older completers are distinctly different (at least on this one dimension).

5–037 Kraas, E., Schuster, H.-P., Baum, P., Schonborn, H., Poeplau, W., & Brodersen, H. Ch. (1971, November 26). [Suicide attempts by poisoning in the aged: Observations on patients of an internal intensive care unit]. Medizinische Klinik, 66, 1653–1660. /*GERMAN*/ (English abstract)

From among 634 patients treated for suicidal poisoning at a medical clinic during a three and one-half year period, 59 cases were 60 years of age or older and were retired. These older individuals were compared to the 575 persons under 60 who were treated for suicidal poisoning during the same period. The characteristic features of suicide by poisoning in the aged were

observed to be: a higher   percentage of   serious attempts,   a
higher   rate   of   complications,   preexisting   organic   disease,
especially malignancy,   and   increased   mortality.   Different
ranges   of   motives   were   found   for   the   younger and older age
groupings also.

5-038   Kuhnert, S. (1981).   [Suicidal cases in   homes   for   the   aged.]
Zeitschrift   fur   Gerontologie,   14(6),   501-507.   /*GERMAN*/
(English abstract) (Abstract: PA, 1982, 68, No. 6024, p. 663)

This   study   found   that   conditions   that   lead   to
institutionalization among   the   elderly   are   similar   to those
associated with high suicide risk in old age.   These   conditions
included both personal factors and life events.

5-039   Kulawik, H., & Decke, D. (1973).   [An analysis   of   223   letters
and messages left behind after completed suicides].   Psychiatria
Clinica,   6(4),   193-210.   /*GERMAN*/   (Abstracts: EM,   1974,
Sect. 32, 29, No. 3631, p. 630;   EM,   1974,   Sect. 20,   17,
No. 2262, p. 379)

5-040   Lauter,   H. (1973).   [Depression   of   old   age: Causes,
epidemiology, nosology].   Aktuelle Gerontologie, 3(5), 247-252.
/*GERMAN*/ (Abstracts: EM,   1974,   Sect. 32,   29,   No. 2638,
p. 459;   EM, 1974, Sect. 20, 17, No. 1796, p. 303)

5-041   Lauter, H. (1974, June).   [Geriatric   psychiatry,   Epidemiologic
aspects of   geriatric   psychiatric   diseases].   Nervenarzt, 45,
277-288.   /*GERMAN*/

5-042   Lemperiere, T., & Jullien, P. (1972, April 21).   [Suicide in the
aged].   Revue du Praticien, 22(12), 1955-1960.   /*FRENCH*/

5-043   Lesson, G. W. (1982).   [Suicide among the elderly   in   Denmark.]
Ugeskrift for Laeger, 144(40), 2965-2968.   /*DANISH*/ (English
abstract)

5-044   Mastrostefano, M. P., Gianturco, F., & Di   Pretoro,   L. (1968).
[Acute poisonings   in   the   aged].   Acta Anaesthesiologica, 19,
Supplement 9, 312+.   /*ITALIAN*/

5-045   Mathe, A. (1967).   [Suicides of the aged].   Vie   Medicale,   48,
91-96.   /*FRENCH*/

5-046   Matsumoto, T. (1980).   [Research on the   psychology   of   suicide
and its primary social causes: Life history analysis of elderly
people   who   have   committed   suicide.]   Otsuma   Joshidaigaku
Kaseigakubu Kiyo, 16, 135-152.   /*JAPANESE*/

5-047   Medvecky, J., Brandebur,   O.,   &   Sestakova, A. (1976).   [An
extraordinary   way   of   suicide].   Ceskoslovenska   Psychiatrie,
72(4), 255-259.   /*CZECH*/ (English   abstract) (Abstract: PA,
1979, 62, No. 11196, p. 1166)

This article presents the case of an 80–year–old woman who attempted suicide by driving a nail into her skull. She had a history of depression and had made one previous attempt.

5-048 Mehne, P. (1977, February). [Cause and incidence of suicides and attempted suicides by patients over 65 years old in psychiatric hospitals]. Aktuelle Gerontologie, 7(2), 105–108. /*GERMAN*/ (English abstract) (Abstracts: EM, 1977, Sect. 20, 20, No. 3473, p. 631; EM, 1977, Sect. 32, 36, No. 3783, p. 700–701)

This study reports the results of a study of 184 suicides and attempted suicides from the case reports of 25 hospitals, including 25 patients who were over 65 years of age. Consideration of nearly 30 variables revealed no significant combination caused by old age and no assessment criteria for suicidal tendencies in hospital patients could be found. The author concluded, however, that suicide risk in hospitals does not increase as a result of lessening restrictions. The author suggests expansion of "hospital suicides" to include the time after discharge.

5-049 Menahem, R. (1972). [Temporal semantic space at different stages of life and its destructuration in suicidal crises]. Annee Psychologique, 72, 353–377. /*FRENCH*/ (English abstract)

5-050 Miketic, B. (1972). [Suicidal behavior and suicide attempts by old people living in a home for the aged]. Anali Zavoda za Mentalno Zdravlje, 4(1), 11–17. /*SERBO–CROATIAN*/ (English summary) (Abstracts: PA, 1975, 53, No. 5631, p. 709; EM, 1973, Sect. 20, 16, No. 1929, p. 316)

This article presents the results of a study of suicidal behavior over a 5–year period in a home for the aged. Of over 400 residents above age 60 (of both sexes), 41 showed some form of suicidal behavior, primarily in the form of verbal communications. Suicidal behavior increased from 3 in 1966 to 13 in 1970. There were 10 actual suicide attempts during the period of study, 8 by drugs, and 2 of the attempts ended in death. Miketic suggests that suicidal behavior and attempts among elderly in homes for the aged have recently increased. Suicidal acts are rare however and only a small number of aged with suicidal ideation will try to commit suicide. The number of suicides compared to the number of attempts are quite small in this population. The author suggests that conflicts that occur in a narrower social environment as well as the personality of the individual are most likely to lead to suicidal tendencies. Chronic frustration is felt to play the main role in such feelings. The major cause of the suicide attempts was seen to be chronic depression.

5-051 Morineau, M. C. (1983, June–July). [Is suicide an important problem in geriatrics?] (Interview). Soins Psychiatrie, p. 45. /*FRENCH*/

5-052 Nezahat, T. (1956). [Note on the Turkish family and the rate of suicide of married people]. Transactions of the third world congress of sociology, 4, 113-115. /*FRENCH*/

5-053 Nick, J., Moinet, A., des Lauriers, A., Guillard, A., & Nicolle, M. (1966). [Suicide due to isolation]. Annales Medico-Psychologiques, 124(1), 5-18. /*FRENCH*/

5-054 Oesterreich, K. (1978). [Crisis intervention in old age]. Therapiewoche, 28(14), 2908-2910. /*GERMAN*/ (Abstract: EM, 1979, Sect. 32, 39, No. 2710, p. 478; EM, 1978, Sect. 20, 21, No. 3206, p. 591)

5-055 Ohara, K. (1961a). [Suicide in old age]. Seishin Shinkeigaku Zasshi, 63, 1253-1268.

Reporting on the suicide rates of older individuals in Japan, the author notes that the old have the highest suicide rate of any age group and that Japan has the highest incidence of late life suicide in the world (see Ruzicka, 1976, reference 4-082, for international data in old age). The author analyzed 1,926 cases of suicide and found that 8.1% were over age 60 (N=156) and 5.5% were over 65 (N=105). The old preferred strangulation and drowning as their suicide methods. They left fewer suicide notes behind than did other age groups and somatic disease was the major factor in the late life suicides.

The author divided a sample of older subjects into two groups, those living in the community and those living in old people's homes, and conducted a survey. Analysis of the responses revealed that significantly more older people living in old people's homes desired to kill themselves in the past (32.3% compared to 9.5% living in the community). The main reasons given for suicide among these elderly old people's home residents were loneliness and family troubles.

5-056 Ohara, K. (1961b). [Suicide of the aged]. Psychiatria et Neurologia Japonica, 63(13), 1253-1268. /*JAPANESE*/

5-057 Ohara, K. (1963). [Suicide in the aged and its counter-measures]. Ronen-byo, 7, 758-765.

5-058 Ohara, K., Okuda, H., Tsuzura, M., & Mashino, H. (1961). [A psychiatric study of the aged with focus on suicide]. Seishin Igaku (Clinical Psychiatry), 3(10), 837-843. /*JAPANESE*/

5-059 Ohara, K., Okuda, Y., Tsuzura, M., & Mashino, H. (1962). [A study on mental health of old age from the viewpoint of suicide]. Yokufuen Chosa Kenkyu Kiyo, 39, 79-87. (English abstract)

5-060 [Old age and death: Repression or conquest? Aging, dying, death, suicide, euthanasia]. (1975). Beschaeftigungtherapie und Rehabilitation, 14(1), 28-30. /*GERMAN*/ (Abstract: EM, 1976,

Sect. 20, 19, No. 933, p. 165)

5-061   Ott, B. (1974, September 27). [Non-psychotic attempted suicide in adults and adolescents]. Medizinische Welt, 25(39), 1545-1548. /*GERMAN*/ (Abstract: EM, 1975, Sect. 32, 32, No. 1798, pp. 305-306)

5-062   Otto, K.-R. (1979). [Prophylaxis of suicide in old age]. Zeitschrift fur Alternsforschung, 34(5), 455-459. /*GERMAN*/ (English summary)

This report focuses on the prevention of suicide among the old, particularly those living alone during Christmas and the end of the year. It is reported that after two weeks of special attention in a hospital the old person feels that they can better handle their life and have a more active outlook on the biological and social circumstances associated with old age.

5-063   Pasquali, L., & Bucher, R. E. (1981). [Suicidal attempts according to sex and age.] Acta Psiquiatrica y Psicologica de America Latina, 27(1), 39-43. /*PORTGUESE*/ (English abstract) (Abstract: PA, 1982, 68, No. 3773, p. 415)

Suicide attempts were analyzed with regard to sex, age, marital status, family relationships, methods, and motives. Canonical analyses found no relationship between the demographic variables with respect to the number, kind, methods, or motives of attempted suicide. A univariate multiple regression analysis, however, indicated that (1) as age increases motives for attempts change from family difficulties predominantly to social and professional problems, and (2) that males made more serious attempts (i.e., their attempts are more planned and employ more lethal means). Age was confounded with sex in this sample (i.e., the male group was older than the female) and therefore it is not clear which characteristic was the better predictor.

5-064   Petrilowitsch, N. (1968). [Problem areas in older persons as reflected in suicidal patients.] In [Problems of psychotherapy among older persons] (2nd ed.). New York: Karger. /*GERMAN*/

5-065   Ravagnan, R., Carassai, P., Vetro, A., & Chiello, A. (1972). [Statistical study on the ages of 3,552 attempted suicides treated at the Policlinico Universitario of Milan during the 5-year period of 1967-1971]. Atti Della Accademia Medica Lombarda, 27(1-4), 42-48. /*ITALIAN*/ (English abstract)

5-066   Reckel, K. (1971). [Peculiarities of suicide in advanced age]. Aktuelle Gerontologie, 1(9), 547-552. /*GERMAN*/ (Abstract: EM, 1973, Sect. 20, 16, No. 705, p. 113)

5-067   Reda, G. C., Rambelli, L., Casini-Nencini, G., & Baldeschi, A. (1957). Il tenatavio di suicidio nei soggetti al di sopra dei 60 anni. In Fourth Congress of the International Association of Gerontology (pp. 231-237). Tito Mattioli,

Fidenze, Vol. IV.   /*ITALIAN*/

5-068   Richert, J., & Classen, C. (1977, December 20).   [Suicidal trend
in the aged: Prevention and therapy of suicide in the   aged   by
the general   practitioner].   ZFA, 53(35), 2211-2216.   /*GERMAN*/

5-069   Robinet,   L. (1934).   [Suicides,   tuberculosis,   senility,
magnesium earths].   Bulletin   de   l'Academie   de Medecine, III,
501-509.   /*FRENCH*/

5-070   Rudolf, G. A. (1973,   October).   [Mental   problems   of   aging].
Oeff Gesundhertswes, 35, Supplement 1, 11-20.   /*GERMAN*/

5-071   Scala, A., Bovo, P. B., Ferraro, G., & Grattagliano,   P. (1977).
[Old people   and   the urban environment: Social and therapeutic
problems].   Ospedale Psichiatrico, 45(4), 360-372.   /*ITALIAN*/
(English abstract) (Abstract: EM, 1979, Sect. 20, 22, No. 1685,
p. 297)

5-072   Schadewaldt, H. (1977,   February).   [Historical   aspects   of
suicide in   the   old   age].   Aktuelle Gerontologie, 7(2), 59-66.
/*GERMAN*/ (English abstract) (Abstract: EM,   1977,   Sect. 20,
20, No. 3469, p. 630)

The author   discusses   suicide   generally   and   old   age suicide
specifically from antiquity   through   the   time   of   Pythagoros,
Aristotle, Cicero,   the   Christian   era   to   the   present.   The
differing beliefs   with   their   sanctions   or   prohibitions   are
discussed at each period.

5-073   Schaub, H. (1955).   [Suicide and suicide attempts   in   the
elderly]. Basal: B. Schwabe.   /*GERMAN*/

5-074   Schindler, B. (1983). [Suicide in old age: Problems of   method
and   methodology   in   studying   acts   of   suicide].
Soziologenkorrespondenz, 9, 203-218.   /*GERMAN*/ (Abstract: SA,
1984, 32, No. 84N6843, pp. 182-183)

The various   forms   of   suicidal   behavior,   both   direct   and
indirect, are discussed with the problems that the latter create
for definition   and   theory highlighted. The author attempts to
classify different types of intention among suicidal elderly and
the social factors that lead to suicide.

5-075   Schlettwein-Gsell, D. (1970, June).   [Self-poisoning in   older
patients]. Hippokrates, 41, 297-298.   /*GERMAN*/

5-076   Schmidt, D. (1977, February).   [Suicides   in   patients of   a
geriatric hospital].   Aktuelle Gerontologie,   7(2), 101-104.
/*GERMAN*/ (English abstract) (Abstract: EM,   1977,   Sect. 20,
No. 3472, pp. 630-631)

The problem of suicide in geriatric hospitals and its prevention
are discussed.

5-077   Schubert, R., Staudacher, H. L., & Haferkamp, G. (1968, January). [Poisoning in the elderly]. Zeitschrift fur Gerontologie, 1(1), 15-20. /*GERMAN*/

5-078   Seidel, K. (1969). [The independent internal dynamics of suicide in the aged]. Social Psychiatry, 9, 42-62. (Bilbiotheca Psychiatria et Neurologia, No. 142) /*GERMAN*/ (English abstract)

A statistical and case study was made of 6913 suicides over an 11 year period in one area (all suicides were studied during that period). The factors peculiarly associated with elderly suicide that resulted from this comprehensive study were: increasing failure of psychophysical capacity, affective changes with age, poor social integration, hypochondriacal and paranoid tendencies, feelings of rapid time passage and nearness to death, loss of that which gives life meaning and value, and restricted social existence of old age.

5-079   Sendbuehler, J. M. (1979). [Certain characteristic features of pre- and post-suicidal states in attempted suicides by aged subjects]. Medecine et Hygiene, 37, 2359-2360. /*FRENCH*/ (Abstract: EM, 1980, Sect. 20, 23, No. 290, p. 47)

A case study of an attempt by an elderly female is presented to illustrate certain components of a serious suicidal state. This woman had an organic cerebral syndrome which probably interfered with her determination to die. Sendbuehler contends that such organic cerebral syndrome is present in 50% of elderly attempters. It is this organic brain syndrome which results in the nonfatalness of the attempt since the old usually die if they attempt suicide. It is suggested that fatal suicidal acts usually require coordination, preparation, determination and consciousness of reality. Organic brain syndromes interfere with these elements.

5-080   Staudacher, H. L. (1970). [Rehabilitation and recidivism with suicide attempts in the aged]. Veroffentlichungen der Deutschen Gesellschaft fur Gerontologie, 4, 313-316.

5-081   Staudacher, H. L. (1971). [Exogenous intoxications in the aged]. Aertzliche Praxis, 23(20), 1152-1159. /*GERMAN*/ (Abstract: EM, 1972, Sect. 20, 15, No. 1569, pp. 255-256)

5-082   Summa, J. D. (1977). [Complications accompanying suicide attempts in old age]. Fortschritte der Medizin, 95 (27), 1729-1736. /*GERMAN*/ (English abstract) (Abstract: EM, 1978, Sect. 20, 21, No. 1447, pp. 268-269)

Summa reports that 11.3% of patients who attempt suicide are over 60 years of age. However, the attempts of the old are more complicated and serious than among the young in cases of medical drug intoxications as the method. Although only 11.3% of all cases, the old comprise 20% of the "grave" suicidal

intoxications and almost 50% of the fatal suicidal
intoxications. The reasons that older persons who use poisons
are more likely to have grave or fatal outcomes are: (a) they
are more likely to be isolated from family and society which
delays proper treatment, and (b) physical changes with old age
complicate the poisoning and its treatment. It is suggested
that the elimination of particularly bromide hypnotics
prescriptions cannot lessen the suicide rate overall, but it
could lower the number of grave, complicated and fatal
intoxications among the elderly.

5-083   Summa, J. D., Platt, D., Maywald, M., & Muhlberg, W. (1982).
[Suicide and old age.] Medizinische Welt, 33(15), 565-569.
/*GERMAN*/

5-084   Swiatecka, G., & Niznikiewicz, J. (1980). [Suicide and
attempted suicide among adults.] Polski Tygodnik Lekarski,
35(29), 1105-1108. /*POLISH*/ (English abstract)

5-085   Takabayashi, T. (1978a). [A case study about the suicide of
aged--Two types of the aged]. Sosharu Waku Kenkyu, 3(3), 37-45.
/*JAPANESE*/

5-086   Takabayashi, T. (1978b). [Some types of suicide among the aged
and their prevention]. Toyo Daigaku Daigakuin Kiyo, 14, 59-72.
/*JAPANESE*/

5-087   Taleghani, M. (1979). Depression et suicide en Haute Normandie.
Revue de Geriatrie, 4, 223-224; 229-233.

5-088   Tanaka, T. (1975, November). [Circumstances leading to suicide
in three aged patients]. Japanese Journal of Nursing, 39(11),
1134-1135. /*JAPANESE*/

5-089   Taragano, F. (1962). [The psychodynamics of day and night
suicide in cerebral arteriosclerosis]. Acta Psiquiatrica y
Psicologica de America Latina, 8(1), 33-36. /*SPANISH*/
(Abstract: PA, 1963, 37, No. 7048, p. 700)

Among patients with cerebral arteriosclerosis who commit
suicide, day suicides are characterized by conscious intent to
die, serious psychotic symptomology, inwardly turned,
unconscious aggression, and regression to magical thinking and
denial of death levels. Night suicides on the other hand, were
most often without suicide intent, had less serious psychosis,
and the suicide was more often an accidental complication.

5-090   Taschev, T., & Roglev, M. (1973). [The fate of adult depressive
patients]. Achiv fur Psychiatrie und Nervenkrankheiten, 217(4),
377-386. (Abstract: EM, 1974, Sect. 32, 29, No. 3624, p. 629)

Case histories of 332 patients who died after experiencing at
least one depressive episode were studied. The authors found
that the majority of depressive patients died between the ages

of 40 and 70. Cerebrovascular disease, as with the population as a whole, was the major cause of death (26.8%), but suicide was next (25.6%). Men predominated the suicides and the highest proportion of suicides was in the 60–70 age group.

5-091   Van Amerongen, P. (1972). [Suicide and suicidal attempt in old age]. Gazette Medicale de France, 79(29), 4841–4847. /*FRENCH*/ (Abstract: EM, 1973, Sect. 20, 16, No. 3836, p. 636)

The author discusses suicide among the old and notes the tremendous determination that usually exists in their attempts. It is suggested that old age suicide is not always the result of chronic mental disease but often occurs in a state of lessened dementia during a psychotic disorder. During this time period the elderly person, to the best of their ability, becomes aware of the possibility of suicide as a way of adapting to their situation of frustration, disillusionment, and physical illness.

5-092   Venzlaff, U. (1980). [The life situation of old people with reference to suicide risk]. Munchener Medizinische Wochenschrift, 122(18), 671–676. /*GERMAN*/

5-093   Vidone, G. (1927). [Contribution to the study of suicide with special regard to age and sex]. Gironale di Psichiatria Clinica e Tecnica Manicomiale, 55, 1–34. /*ITALIAN*/

5-094   Wachtler, C. (1982). [Suicide attempts in old age: A follow-up study.] Aktuelle Gerontologie, 12(2), 64–66. /*RUSSIAN*/ (English abstract)

5-095   Wachtler, C. (1984). [Suicidal behavior of elderly.] Psychiatrische Praxis, 11, 14–19. /*GERMAN*/ (English abstract)

5-096   Wiendieck, G. (1970a, March). [Social psychologic factors in old age suicide]. Nervenarzt, 41, 220–223. /*GERMAN*/

5-097   Wiendieck, G. (1970b). [Social determinants of suicide in the aged]. Veroffentlichungen der Deutschen Gessellschaft fur Gerontologie, 4, 125–131.

5-098   Wiendieck, G. (1973). [The psychosocial determination of suicide in old age]. Aktuelle Gerontologie, 3(5), 271–274. /*GERMAN*/ (Abstracts: EM, 1974, Sect. 20, 17, No. 1797, p. 303; EM, 1974, Sect. 32, 29, No. 2648, p. 460)

This article suggests that suicidal behavior is the result of ambivalent intrapsychic forces which decide between the avoidance and choice of suicide. To the degree to which one feels that solutions to problems will be unsatisfactory, the component toward choice will be stronger and suicide more likely. It is suggested that aging increases the probability that factors which favor suicide might occur and lessens the likelihood that satisfactory solutions to problems may be found. Therefore the probability of lethal suicidal behavior increases in old age and this tendency is supported by societal norms that suggest that suicide is more comprehensible among the old than among younger persons. Therefore, norms facilitate suicide decisions in old age.

5-099   Yampey, N. (1972). [Cultural factors in the present prevalence of suicide among older persons]. In R. E. Litman (Ed.), <u>Proceedings: Sixth International Conference for Suicide Prevention</u> (pp. 441-448), Mexico, D.F., Mexico, December 5-8, 1971. Ann Arbor, MI: Edwards Brothers, Inc. /*SPANISH*/

5-100   Zemek, P., & Drdkova, S. (1975, October). [Some possibilities of prevention in elderly people suicide with regard to aid by telephone]. <u>Sbornik Lekarsky</u>, <u>77</u>(10), 308-312. /*CZECH*/ (English abstract)

DEMOGRAPHIC APPENDIX

Official suicide data are available in published form in several sources. Although the existing data have omissions and limitations (as pointed out in Chapter 2), they provide the best information available regarding the levels of suicide among the old and other demographic groups. The quality and accuracy of official suicide data have often been questioned (e.g., Atkinson, 1978, Chapter 3; Douglas, 1968, Chapter 12). Other evidence, however, has been presented which suggests that although suicide rates are most likely underestimates, they contain little systematic bias (Sainsbury & Barraclough, 1968; Sainsbury & Jenkins, 1982). In fact, official figures are our only consistent source of nationwide suicide data. Despite their flaws, they are almost certainly the most conservative estimates of the numbers which actually occur (Hatton, Valente, & Rink, 1977).

Below are listed sources of official suicide data for the United States and some sources of international data as well as the references in which the tables and figures that follow may be found or from which they were compiled. Figures displaying the trends over time in methods of suicide by age, sex, and race may be found in McIntosh and Santos (1985–86, reference 4–063) for the years 1960 to 1978.

REFERENCES NOT FOUND IN ANNOTATIONS

Atkinson, J. M. (1978). Discovering suicide: Studies in the social organization of sudden death. Pittsburgh, PA: University of Pittsburgh Press.

Douglas, J. D. (1968). The social meanings of suicide. Princeton, NJ: Princeton University Press.

Hatton, C. L., Valente, S. M., & Rink, A. (1977). Variables in suicide statistics. In C. L. Hatton, S. M. Valente, & A. Rink (Eds.), Suicide: Assessment and intervention (pp. 133–138). New York: Appleton-Century-Crofts.

Sainsbury, P., & Barraclough, B. (1968). Differences between suicide rates. Nature, 220, 1252.

Sainsbury, P., & Jenkins, J. S. (1982). The accuracy of officially reported suicide statistics for purposes of epidemiological research. Journal of Epidemiology and Community Health, 36, 43–48.

SOURCES OF OFFICIAL SUICIDE DATA

A-001   Grove, Robert D., & Hetzel, Alice M. (1968)   Vital statistics
        rates in the United States 1940–1960. Washington, D.C.: United
        States Government Printing Office.

A-002   Linder, Forrest E., & Grove, Robert D. (1943). Vital statistics
        in the United States 1900 1940. Washington, D.C.: United
        States Government Printing Office.

A-003   Massey, James T. (1967). Suicide in the United States,
        1950–1964. Vital and Health Statistics Series 20, No. 5,
        Public Health Service Publication No. 1000.

A-004   National Center for Health Statistics. Annual volumes of Vital
        Statistics of the United States, Parts I & II (for 1936–1949
        data), Volume II (for 1950–1959 data), Volume II--Mortality,
        Parts A & B (for 1960-1980 data currently). [Prior to 1937,
        published data for 1900–1936 may be found in Mortality
        Statistics.] Washington, D.C.: United States Government
        Printing Office.

A-005   National Center for Health Statistics. (1984a, June 22).
        Advance report of final mortality statistics, 1981. NCHS
        Monthly Vital Statistics Report, 33(3, Supplement).

A-006   National Center for Health Statistics. (1984b, December 20).
        Advance report of final mortality statistics, 1982. NCHS
        Monthly Vital Statistics Report, 33(9, Supplement).

A-007   National Center for Health Statistics. (1985, September 26).
        Advance report of final mortality statistics, 1983. NCHS
        Monthly Vital Statistics Report, 34(6, Supplement(2)).

A-008   National Office of Vital Statistics. (1956, August 22). Death
        rates by age, race, and sex: United States, 1900–1953:
        Suicide. Vital and Health Statistics--Special Report, 43(30).

A-009   United Nations. Annual volumes of Demographic Yearbook. New
        York: United Nations.

        International statistics.

A-010   World Health Organization. Annual volumes of World health
        statistics annual. Geneva, Switzerland: World Health
        Organization.

        International statistics.

SOURCES OF TABLES AND FIGURES

Table 1 is taken from compilations made in:
McIntosh, J. L. (1980). A study of suicide among United States racial
    minorities based on official statistics: The influence of age, sex,
    and other variables (University of Notre Dame, 1980). <u>Dissertation
    Abstracts International</u>, <u>41</u>,   1135B.   (University   Microfilms
    No. 8020965)

Table 2 appears in:
McIntosh, J. L. (1985, April 20). <u>Middle age suicide: Sex and race
    differences</u>. Paper presented at the annual meeting of the American
    Association of Suicidology, Toronto, Ontario, Canada.

Table 3 and Table 4 appear in:
McIntosh, J. L., & Jewell, B. L. (1984, May 3). <u>Sex difference trends
    in completed suicide</u>. Paper presented at the annual meeting of the
    American Association of Suicidology, Anchorage, AK.

Table 5 appears in both of the following references:
McIntosh, J. L., & Jewell, B. L. (1984, May 3). <u>Sex difference trends
    in completed suicide</u>. Paper presented at the annual meeting of the
    American Association of Suicidology, Anchorage, AK.

McIntosh, J. L. (1985, April 20). <u>Middle age suicide: Sex and race
    differences</u>. Paper presented at the annual meeting of the American
    Association of Suicidology, Toronto, Ontario, Canada.

Table 6 data are taken from:
Annual volumes of the <u>Vital Statistics of the United States</u> for the
    years 1960–1980 (reference A–004) and for 1981, 1982, and 1983 from
    NCHS (references A–005, A–006, & A–007, respectively).   Some rates
    have been calculated from data in these sources and the population
    estimate sources listed at the end of Table 1.

Figures 1–5 appear in:
McIntosh, J. L. (1984). Components of the decline in elderly suicide:
    Suicide among the young-old and old-old by race and sex. <u>Death
    Education</u>, <u>8</u>(Supplement), 113–124. [reference 4–059]

Table 1
Contribution of the Elderly to Suicide and Population, 1900–1983

	Population (in thousands)			Suicides				
	No.			No.			Rates (per 100,000)	
Year	Total	Aged	% Aged	Total	Aged	% Aged	Total	Aged
1983	234023	27474	11.74	28295	5284	18.67	12.09	19.23
1982	231822	26861	11.59	28242	4919	17.42	12.18	18.31
1981	229542	26259	11.44	27596	4478	16.23	12.02	17.05
1980	227236	25709	11.31	26869	4537	16.89	11.82	17.65
1979	224567	25134	11.19	27206	4701	17.28	12.11	18.70
1978	222095	24502	11.03	27294	4783	17.52	12.29	19.52
1977	219760	23892	10.87	28681	4763	16.60	13.05	19.94
1976	217563	23278	10.70	26832	4549	16.95	12.33	19.54
1975	215465	22696	10.53	27063	4436	16.39	12.56	19.55
1974	213342	22061	10.34	25683	4221	16.43	12.04	19.13
1973	211357	21525	10.18	25118	4326	17.22	11.88	20.10
1972	209284	21020	10.04	25004	4382	17.53	11.95	20.85
1971	206827	20561	9.94	24092	4298	17.84	11.65	20.90
1970	203984	20107	9.86	23480	4171	17.76	11.51	20.74
1969	201385	19680	9.77	22364	4123	18.44	11.11	20.95
1968	199399	19365	9.71	21372	3852	18.02	10.72	19.89
1967	197457	19071	9.66	21325	3828	17.95	10.80	20.07
1966	195576	18755	9.59	21281	4161	19.55	10.88	22.19
1965	193526	18451	9.53	21507	4140	19.25	11.11	22.44
1964	191141	18127	9.48	20588	4078	19.81	10.77	22.50
1963	188483	17778	9.43	20825	4109	19.73	11.05	23.11
1962	185771	17457	9.40	20207	4144	20.51	10.88	23.74
1961	182992	17089	9.34	18999	3966	20.87	10.38	23.21
1960	179979	16675	9.26	19041	4059	21.32	10.58	24.34
1959	177135	16248	9.17	18633	4169	22.37	10.52	25.66
1958	174149	15806	9.08	18519	4079	22.03	10.63	25.81
1957	171187	15388	8.99	16632	3775	22.70	9.72	24.53
1956	168088	14938	8.89	16727	3859	23.07	9.95	25.83
1955	165069	14525	8.80	16760	3741	22.32	10.15	25.76
1954	161884	14076	8.70	16356	3545	21.67	10.10	25.18
1953	158956	13617	8.57	15947	3565	22.36	10.03	26.18
1952	156393	13203	8.44	15567	3490	22.42	9.95	26.43
1951	153982	12803	8.31	15909	3502	22.01	10.33	27.35
1950	151868	12397	8.16	17145	3654	21.31	11.29	29.47

CONTINUED

Table 1 (continued)
Contribution of the Elderly to Suicide and Population, 1900–1983

	Population (in thousands)			Suicides				
	No.		%	No.		%	Rates (per 100,000)	
Year	Total	Aged	Aged	Total	Aged	Aged	Total	Aged
1949	148665	11921	8.02	16993	3463	20.38	11.43	29.05
1948	146093	11538	7.90	16354	3243	19.83	11.19	28.11
1947	143446	11185	7.80	16538	3319	20.07	11.53	29.67
1946	140054	10828	7.73	16152	2945	18.23	11.53	27.20
1945	132481	10494	7.92	14782	2858	19.33	11.16	27.23
1944	132885	10147	7.64	13231	2549	19.27	9.96	25.12
1943	134245	9867	7.35	13725	2692	19.61	10.22	27.28
1942	133920	9583	7.16	16117	2797	17.35	12.03	29.19
1941	133121	9288	6.98	17102	2934	17.16	12.85	31.59
1940	131669	8968	6.81	18907	2999	15.86	14.36	33.44
1939	130880	8747	6.68	18511	2981	16.10	14.14	34.08
1938	129825	8480	6.53	19802	2931	14.80	15.25	34.56
1937	128825	8225	6.38	19294	2901	15.04	14.98	35.27
1936	128053	7986	6.24	18294	2813	15.38	14.29	35.22
1935	127250	7751	6.09	18214	2806	15.41	14.31	36.20
1934	126374	7520	5.95	18828	3033	16.11	14.90	40.33
1933	125579	7301	5.81	19993	3307	16.54	15.92	45.30
1932	118904	6842	5.75	20646	3347	16.21	17.36	48.92
1931	118149	6649	5.63	19807	3087	15.59	16.76	46.43
1930	117238	6458	5.51	18323	2684	14.65	15.63	41.56
1929	115317	6212	5.39	16045	2507	15.62	13.91	40.36
1928	113636	6022	5.30	15390	2394	15.56	13.54	39.75
1927	107085	5665	5.29	14096	2092	14.84	13.16	36.93
1926	103823	5437	5.24	13082	2073	15.85	12.60	38.13
1925	102032	5264	5.16	12495	1826	14.61	12.25	34.69
1924	99318	5053	5.09	12061	1649	13.67	12.14	32.63
1923	96788	4857	5.02	11287	1570	13.91	11.66	32.32
1922	92703	4543	4.90	11053	1526	13.81	11.92	33.59
1921	87814	4286	4.88	11136	1394	12.52	12.68	32.52
1920	86079	4161	4.83	8959	1156	12.90	10.41	27.78
1919	83158	4060	4.88	9732	1257	12.92	11.70	30.96
1918	79008	3898	4.93	9937	1191	11.99	12.58	30.55
1917	70235	3427	4.88	10056	1228	12.21	14.32	35.83
1916	66971	3258	4.86	10162	1243	12.23	15.17	38.15
1915	61895	3047	4.92	11216	1262	11.25	18.12	41.42

CONTINUED

Table 1 (continued)
Contribution of the Elderly to Suicide and Population, 1900–1983

	Population (in thousands)			Suicides					
	No.			No.			Rates (per 100,000)		
Year	Total	Aged	% Aged	Total	Aged	% Aged	Total	Aged	
1914	60963	2985	4.90	10933	1118	10.23	17.93	37.45	
1913	58157	2823	4.85	9988	1027	10.28	17.17	36.38	
1912	54848	2665	4.86	9656	1006	10.42	17.61	37.75	
1911	53930	2610	4.84	9622	986	10.25	17.84	37.78	
1910	47470	2313	4.87	8590	930	10.83	18.10	40.21	
1909	44224	2167	4.90	8402	877	10.44	19.00	40.47	
1908	38635	1861	4.82	8332	795	9.54	21.57	42.72	
1907	34553	1670	4.83	6745	695	10.30	19.52	41.62	
1906	33782	1629	4.82	5853	637	10.88	17.33	39.10	
1905	21768	1107	5.09	5438	581	10.68	24.98	52.48	
1904	21332	1082	5.07	4912	493	10.04	23.03	45.56	
1903	20943	1061	5.07	4510	435	9.65	21.53	41.00	
1902	20583	1042	5.06	4054	432	10.66	19.70	41.46	
1901	20237	1024	5.06	3824	401	10.49	18.90	39.16	
1900	19965	1010	5.06	3534	392	11.09	17.70	38.81	

Sources: Population: 1980–1983:   U.S. Bureau of the Census (1985), Current Population Reports [CPR], Series P–25, No. 965; 1970–1979:   Estimates consistent with the 1980 census, U.S. Bureau of Census (1982), CPR, No. 917 [Note: 1970–1979 rates have been recalculated and may differ from rates published in Vital Statistics of the U.S. due to differing population estimates.]; 1950–1969:   U.S. Bureau of the Census, CPR, Nos. 643, 614, 519, & 310;   1933–1949:   Grove & Hetzel (1968, reference A–001);   1900–1932:   Linder & Grove (1943, reference A–002).
Suicide: 1983:   National Center for Health Statistics (NCHS) (1985, reference A–007);   1982:   NCHS (1984b, reference A–006);   1981:   NCHS (1984a, reference A–005);   1936–1980:   NCHS, Vital Statistics of the U.S. for year indicated (reference A–004);   1900–1936: NCHS, Mortality Statistics for year indicated (reference A–004).
Rates & Percentages: Computed from suicide and population figures.

Note: Elderly/Aged = 65 years of age and over.

Table 2
Suicide Rates by 10-Year Age Groups, 1933–1983

Year	Age Groups					
	15–24	25–34	35–44	45–54	55–64	65+
1983	11.9	15.8	14.6	16.2	16.5	19.2
1982	12.1	16.0	15.3	16.6	16.9	18.3
1981	12.3	16.3	15.9	16.1	16.4	17.1
1980	12.3	16.0	15.4	15.9	15.9	17.7
1979	12.7	16.8	15.5	16.5	17.0	19.1
1978	12.4	16.7	15.8	17.1	18.1	19.9
1977	13.6	17.7	16.8	18.9	19.4	20.3
1976	11.7	15.9	16.3	19.2	20.0	19.8
1975	11.8	16.4	17.4	20.1	20.0	19.8
1974	10.9	15.7	16.8	19.6	19.7	19.3
1973	10.6	14.9	16.4	19.5	20.3	20.3
1972	10.2	14.7	16.8	19.9	21.4	21.0
1971	9.4	13.7	17.2	19.8	21.6	21.0
1970	8.8	14.1	16.9	20.0	21.4	20.8
1969	8.0	12.9	16.6	19.4	21.3	21.0
1968	7.1	12.0	16.1	19.7	21.5	19.9
1967	7.0	12.4	16.6	19.5	22.4	20.1
1966	6.4	12.3	15.8	20.0	22.9	22.2
1965	6.2	12.2	16.7	20.9	23.7	22.4
1964	6.0	11.8	15.5	20.5	22.6	22.5
1963	6.0	11.8	16.0	21.1	23.6	23.1
1962	5.7	11.3	15.0	21.0	23.7	23.7
1961	5.1	10.3	14.4	20.3	23.1	23.2
1960	5.2	10.0	14.2	20.7	23.7	24.3
1959	4.9	9.9	13.6	19.8	24.3	25.7
1958	4.8	9.8	.13.7	20.7	24.1	25.8
1957	4.0	8.7	12.7	18.2	22.4	24.5
1956	4.0	8.5	12.1	18.5	24.2	25.8
1955	4.1	8.4	12.3	19.6	24.8	25.8
1954	4.2	8.7	12.5	19.3	23.9	25.2
1953	4.4	8.5	12.6	18.7	22.4	26.2
1952	4.2	8.5	12.4	18.3	22.5	26.4
1951	4.4	8.6	13.3	18.8	23.2	27.4
1950	4.5	9.1	14.3	20.9	26.8	29.5
1949	4.6	8.8	15.1	20.6	27.6	29.1
1948	4.8	9.0	14.5	20.7	26.0	28.1
1947	4.6	9.4	15.1	20.7	26.7	29.7
1946	5.2	9.9	15.3	20.7	25.9	27.2
1945	4.7	10.3	15.0	19.2	23.5	27.2
1944	4.3	9.1	13.4	17.1	21.5	25.1
1943	4.5	9.0	13.1	17.4	23.5	27.3
1942	5.1	11.5	16.1	21.1	28.0	29.2
1941	5.7	12.4	17.1	23.1	29.4	31.6
1940	6.1	13.5	19.4	27.7	34.3	33.4
1939	5.9	12.9	18.9	28.2	34.4	34.1
1938	6.7	14.5	21.0	30.7	37.5	34.6
1937	6.9	14.4	20.7	30.1	35.5	35.3
1936	6.9	14.5	19.7	27.6	34.1	35.2
1935	7.1	14.3	19.0	28.6	34.9	36.2
1934	7.4	14.5	19.9	29.6	37.2	40.3
1933	7.2	13.9	21.3	33.2	43.0	45.3

Table 3
Suicide Rates Per 100,000 Population by Sex and Age Groups, 1933–1980

Year	15–24		25–34		35–44		45–54		55–64		65+	
	M	F	M	F	M	F	M	F	M	F	M	F
1980	20.2	4.3	25.0	7.1	22.5	8.5	22.9	9.4	24.5	8.4	34.8	6.0
1979	20.4	4.9	26.1	7.7	21.9	9.3	22.7	10.7	25.3	9.6	36.7	7.0
1978	20.0	4.7	25.5	8.1	21.9	10.1	23.4	11.2	27.5	9.7	38.0	7.4
1977	21.8	5.3	26.6	9.0	23.7	10.3	25.6	12.6	29.2	10.5	38.4	7.8
1976	18.5	4.8	23.6	8.4	22.8	10.2	26.2	12.7	29.8	11.1	37.2	7.8
1975	18.9	4.8	24.4	8.6	23.5	11.6	27.9	12.7	30.2	11.0	36.8	8.0
1974	17.1	4.6	23.3	8.4	22.8	11.1	26.6	13.0	30.2	10.3	36.7	7.2
1973	17.0	4.3	21.9	8.1	21.8	11.3	26.9	12.6	30.5	11.2	38.0	7.8
1972	15.7	4.7	20.9	8.8	22.2	11.6	28.0	12.4	31.5	12.4	39.4	7.9
1971	14.1	4.7	19.0	8.6	22.3	12.3	26.7	13.4	32.8	11.7	38.8	8.3
1970	13.5	4.2	19.8	8.6	22.1	11.9	27.9	12.6	32.7	11.4	38.4	8.1
1969	12.3	3.8	18.2	7.8	21.7	11.8	27.0	12.3	32.7	11.0	38.7	8.0
1968	10.9	3.4	17.2	7.1	22.0	10.6	27.3	12.5	33.6	10.6	37.5	6.9
1967	10.5	3.5	17.2	7.6	22.9	10.7	27.5	12.1	34.4	11.5	36.2	8.0
1966	9.7	3.1	17.3	7.6	21.6	10.4	28.5	12.0	36.2	10.8	40.8	8.1
1965	9.4	3.0	17.2	7.4	22.6	11.1	29.4	12.8	37.1	11.3	40.6	8.5
1964	9.2	2.8	16.9	7.0	21.3	10.1	29.9	11.6	36.1	10.2	40.8	8.2
1963	9.0	3.1	16.6	7.2	22.4	9.9	30.8	11.9	37.3	10.9	42.0	8.2
1962	8.5	2.9	15.9	6.8	21.5	8.8	30.9	11.5	37.0	10.4	43.6	7.8
1961	7.9	2.3	14.9	5.8	21.2	7.8	30.9	10.0	37.4	9.7	42.0	7.9
1960	8.2	2.2	14.7	5.5	21.0	7.7	31.6	10.2	38.1	10.2	43.7	8.3
1959	7.7	2.1	14.4	5.4	20.5	7.0	31.0	8.8	39.4	10.1	46.5	8.3
1958	7.4	2.3	14.2	5.6	21.1	6.7	32.1	9.7	39.6	9.4	47.0	8.1
1957	6.4	1.8	12.7	4.8	19.1	6.6	28.6	8.0	35.9	9.6	45.2	7.1
1956	6.3	1.9	12.7	4.5	18.2	6.3	28.3	9.0	39.1	9.9	46.9	7.9
1955	6.3	2.0	12.4	4.6	18.8	6.1	29.7	9.6	40.3	9.8	45.9	8.5
1954	6.7	1.8	13.4	4.3	18.9	6.3	31.0	7.7	39.2	9.0	45.6	7.5
1953	6.6	2.3	12.7	4.5	19.5	6.0	29.3	8.3	36.4	8.7	47.7	7.4
1952	6.6	2.0	12.4	4.7	18.5	6.4	27.9	8.7	36.5	8.7	47.7	7.8
1951	6.6	2.3	12.6	4.8	19.5	7.2	28.6	9.1	37.6	8.8	49.0	8.3
1950	6.5	2.6	13.4	4.9	21.3	7.5	32.0	9.9	43.6	9.9	52.2	9.3
1949	6.7	2.5	13.0	4.8	22.7	7.6	31.6	9.6	44.3	10.8	51.5	8.8
1948	6.6	2.9	12.9	5.2	20.8	8.3	31.5	9.9	42.0	9.9	49.2	8.9
1947	6.6	2.7	13.2	5.7	22.1	8.3	30.5	10.9	43.0	10.2	51.1	10.0
1946	7.4	3.2	14.2	5.9	21.9	8.7	30.3	11.0	40.4	11.2	46.6	9.3
1945	7.4	2.9	15.9	6.4	21.8	8.7	27.2	11.0	36.2	10.6	46.0	9.8
1944	6.0	3.1	13.3	5.7	18.7	8.3	24.2	9.8	32.0	10.8	42.2	9.2
1943	6.3	3.0	12.9	5.6	18.5	7.8	24.5	10.0	35.0	11.6	45.9	9.8
1942	7.0	3.2	16.6	6.8	23.8	8.6	30.9	11.0	44.3	11.2	50.0	9.6
1941	7.5	3.9	17.5	7.5	24.8	9.4	33.8	11.9	46.4	11.8	55.0	9.4
1940	8.4	3.8	19.1	8.1	28.2	10.6	41.6	13.1	55.3	12.3	56.9	11.0
1939	8.0	3.8	18.8	7.2	27.5	10.1	42.1	13.4	54.8	12.9	58.7	10.4
1938	9.0	4.4	20.9	8.2	31.1	10.8	47.0	13.3	60.2	13.4	59.8	10.1
1937	9.0	4.9	20.4	8.5	30.4	10.7	45.5	13.7	56.1	13.6	61.0	10.2
1936	8.8	4.8	19.7	9.3	29.0	10.1	41.9	12.4	54.4	12.6	60.7	10.3
1935	9.0	5.2	19.7	9.1	27.5	10.2	44.1	12.0	55.5	13.1	62.8	10.0
1934	9.2	5.5	20.3	8.7	29.2	10.4	45.0	12.9	60.1	12.7	71.0	10.0
1933	8.8	5.7	19.4	8.4	31.6	10.5	52.8	12.0	70.2	13.9	80.3	10.5

Table 4
Ratio of Male to Female Suicide Rates by Age Groups, 1933–1980

	Age Groups					
Year	15–24	25–34	35–44	45–54	55–64	65+
1980	4.70	3.52	2.65	2.44	2.92	5.80
1979	4.16	3.39	2.35	2.12	2.64	5.24
1978	4.26	3.15	2.17	2.09	2.84	5.14
1977	4.11	2.96	2.30	2.03	2.78	4.92
1976	3.85	2.81	2.24	2.06	2.68	4.77
1975	3.94	2.84	2.03	2.20	2.75	4.60
1974	3.72	2.77	2.05	2.05	2.93	5.10
1973	3.95	2.70	1.93	2.13	2.72	4.87
1972	3.34	2.37	1.91	2.26	2.54	4.99
1971	3.00	2.21	1.81	1.99	2.80	4.67
1970	3.21	2.30	1.86	2.21	2.87	4.74
1969	3.24	2.33	1.84	2.20	2.97	4.84
1968	3.21	2.42	2.08	2.18	3.17	5.43
1967	3.00	2.26	2.14	2.27	2.99	4.53
1966	3.13	2.28	2.08	2.38	3.35	5.04
1965	3.13	2.32	2.04	2.30	3.28	4.78
1964	3.29	2.41	2.11	2.58	3.54	4.98
1963	2.90	2.31	2.26	2.59	3.42	5.12
1962	2.93	2.34	2.44	2.69	3.56	5.59
1961	3.43	2.57	2.72	3.09	3.86	5.32
1960	3.73	2.67	2.73	3.10	3.74	5.27
1959	3.67	2.67	2.93	3.52	3.90	5.60
1958	3.22	2.54	3.15	3.31	4.21	5.80
1957	3.56	2.65	2.89	3.58	3.74	6.37
1956	3.32	2.82	2.89	3.14	3.95	5.94
1955	3.15	2.70	3.08	3.09	4.11	5.40
1954	3.72	3.12	3.00	4.03	4.36	6.08
1953	2.87	2.82	3.25	3.53	4.18	6.45
1952	3.30	2.64	2.89	3.21	4.20	6.12
1951	2.87	2.63	2.71	3.14	4.27	5.90
1950	2.50	2.73	2.84	3.23	4.40	5.61
1949	2.68	2.71	2.99	3.29	4.10	5.85
1948	2.28	2.48	2.51	3.18	4.24	5.53
1947	2.44	2.32	2.66	2.80	4.22	5.11
1946	2.31	2.41	2.52	2.75	3.61	5.01
1945	2.55	2.48	2.51	2.47	3.42	4.69
1944	1.94	2.33	2.25	2.47	2.96	4.59
1943	2.10	2.30	2.37	2.45	3.02	4.68
1942	2.19	2.44	2.77	2.81	3.96	5.21
1941	1.92	2.33	2.64	2.84	3.93	5.85
1940	2.21	2.36	2.66	3.18	4.50	5.17
1939	2.11	2.61	2.72	3.14	4.25	5.64
1938	2.05	2.55	2.88	3.53	4.49	5.92
1937	1.84	2.40	2.84	3.32	4.13	5.98
1936	1.83	2.12	2.87	3.38	4.32	5.89
1935	1.73	2.16	2.70	3.68	4.24	6.28
1934	1.67	2.33	2.81	3.49	4.73	7.10
1933	1.54	2.31	3.01	4.40	5.05	7.65

Table 5
Suicide Rates by Race and 10-Year Age Groups, 1933–1980

Year	15–24		25–34		35–44		45–54		55–64		65+	
	W	NW	W	NW	W	NW	W	NW	W	NW	W	NW
1980	13.1	8.2	16.5	12.4	16.3	9.3	17.0	7.6	17.0	6.9	28.6	6.3
1979	13.1	10.1	17.1	15.0	16.2	10.3	17.7	8.1	18.0	8.3	20.2	7.9
1978	13.0	8.9	17.1	13.9	16.6	10.3	18.3	8.6	19.3	6.9	21.2	7.0
1977	14.3	9.6	18.0	15.5	17.8	10.0	20.3	8.2	20.5	8.5	21.7	6.6
1976	12.1	9.3	16.2	14.0	17.2	10.2	20.5	8.6	21.3	7.2	21.0	8.0
1975	12.3	9.1	16.6	14.8	18.4	9.9	21.5	8.4	21.4	7.5	21.1	6.8
1974	11.4	8.3	16.0	13.9	17.8	9.5	21.0	7.7	21.0	7.6	20.4	7.9
1973	10.9	8.9	15.1	13.3	17.4	9.5	20.8	7.9	21.6	8.0	21.5	7.0
1972	10.1	11.0	15.0	12.7	17.7	10.0	21.3	8.2	22.9	7.5	22.4	6.4
1971	9.6	8.4	13.9	11.9	18.1	10.4	21.2	7.1	23.1	7.4	22.3	7.5
1970	9.0	7.6	14.4	12.2	18.1	8.1	21.2	9.0	23.1	6.1	22.1	6.9
1969	8.1	6.9	13.1	11.6	17.5	9.8	20.7	7.6	22.8	6.2	22.2	7.6
1968	7.3	5.6	12.4	9.6	17.2	8.0	21.0	7.7	23.0	7.1	21.1	7.1
1967	7.1	6.1	12.5	11.4	17.6	9.1	20.9	7.3	23.8	8.1	21.3	6.5
1966	6.5	5.7	12.4	11.7	16.9	6.9	21.3	8.5	24.3	8.8	23.5	8.0
1965	6.2	5.8	12.6	9.5	17.6	9.1	22.2	8.6	25.2	8.2	23.7	7.9
1964	6.1	4.9	12.1	10.0	16.4	8.1	21.9	7.4	24.1	8.0	23.9	6.8
1963	6.2	5.0	12.2	10.0	17.1	9.1	22.8	7.9	25.4	7.4	23.5	9.7
1962	5.8	5.2	11.8	8.4	16.1	8.1	22.7	7.7	25.3	9.1	24.4	8.4
1961	5.1	4.7	10.4	9.4	15.2	7.5	21.6	8.2	24.5	9.0	24.5	7.6
1960	5.4	3.4	10.3	7.9	14.9	8.3	22.1	7.9	25.0	10.0	25.7	7.9
1959	5.0	4.3	10.0	8.7	14.4	6.7	21.0	8.2	25.7	9.4	27.0	9.3
1958	5.0	3.5	10.0	7.8	14.5	7.3	22.1	7.8	25.5	9.0	27.3	7.8
1957	4.1	3.4	8.8	7.4	13.4	6.3	19.4	6.4	23.7	7.9	25.8	9.1
1956	4.1	3.4	8.8	6.4	12.8	6.6	19.8	6.4	25.6	7.7	27.5	6.2
1955	4.1	4.0	8.7	6.0	13.1	5.5	20.9	6.6	26.3	7.6	27.3	6.6
1954	4.3	3.4	8.9	7.4	13.3	6.1	20.5	7.1	25.3	7.5	26.7	7.5
1953	4.6	3.0	8.8	5.8	13.4	5.8	19.9	7.2	23.7	7.0	27.7	7.9
1952	4.4	2.7	8.7	6.5	13.2	5.5	19.6	5.7	23.6	8.3	28.1	5.8
1951	4.5	3.7	8.8	6.4	14.0	6.6	20.0	6.8	24.4	7.5	29.1	6.4
1950	4.7	3.4	9.4	6.3	15.2	6.6	22.3	7.9	28.3	9.1	31.3	7.1
1949	4.8	3.1	9.1	6.0	16.0	6.8	22.0	7.1	29.1	9.4	30.5	8.7
1948	4.9	3.3	9.3	6.0	15.3	7.1	22.0	8.1	27.7	6.0	29.6	7.4
1947	4.7	3.8	9.8	5.9	16.1	6.6	22.2	5.5	28.3	7.8	31.3	7.7
1946	5.4	3.6	10.4	6.0	16.4	5.7	22.1	6.6	27.4	7.7	28.8	6.1
1945	4.9	3.4	10.9	5.5	16.1	5.4	20.5	5.4	25.1	5.3	28.7	6.9
1944	4.5	2.8	9.6	4.5	14.4	4.5	18.2	4.9	22.8	6.3	26.6	4.8
1943	4.7	3.1	9.6	4.5	14.1	4.4	18.6	4.2	24.9	6.3	28.9	4.2
1942	5.2	3.9	12.1	6.5	17.3	6.2	22.6	5.1	29.7	8.2	30.9	4.9
1941	6.0	3.8	13.2	6.3	18.3	6.0	24.5	7.8	31.2	7.2	33.3	6.9
1940	6.4	4.2	14.2	7.3	20.8	6.7	29.4	9.2	36.4	7.3	35.3	7.3
1939	6.2	3.3	13.7	6.5	20.2	7.0	30.0	8.6	36.4	7.3	36.1	6.6
1938	7.0	4.1	15.3	7.5	22.5	7.8	32.7	8.7	39.4	11.2	36.6	7.3
1937	7.3	3.9	15.2	7.6	22.1	8.3	32.1	8.7	37.4	10.0	37.3	7.1
1936	7.1	4.2	15.4	7.0	21.0	7.9	29.6	6.9	35.9	10.8	37.2	6.9
1935	7.4	4.3	15.0	8.4	20.1	8.4	30.6	8.3	36.7	10.7	38.2	6.3
1934	7.6	5.2	15.2	8.4	21.3	7.7	31.6	8.8	39.2	10.5	42.4	8.7
1933	7.5	4.9	14.6	7.4	22.5	9.8	35.4	10.9	45.5	9.0	47.7	8.9

Table 6
Suicide Rates Among Elderly Age Groupings

BOTH SEXES COMBINED

YEAR	55–9	60–4	55–64	65–9	70–4	65–74	75+	75–9	80–4	75–84	85+
1983	–	–	16.5	–	–	17.7	21.5	–	–	22.3	19.0
1982	–	–	16.9	–	–	17.4	19.8	–	–	20.3	17.6
1981	–	–	16.4	–	–	16.2	18.4	–	–	18.6	17.7
1980	16.3	15.5	15.9	16.2	17.8	16.9	19.0	19.6	18.3	19.1	19.2
1979	16.6	17.5	17.0	17.6	18.2	17.9	21.0	23.1	21.3	22.4	16.9
1978	17.8	18.6	18.1	18.0	20.0	18.8	21.6	23.1	21.8	22.6	18.6
1977	19.3	19.4	19.4	19.1	21.4	20.1	20.5	22.5	20.2	21.5	17.3
1976	20.4	19.4	20.0	19.1	20.2	19.5	20.3	20.9	20.5	20.8	18.9
1975	20.6	19.4	20.0	19.3	20.2	19.7	20.0	21.2	19.6	20.6	18.1
1974	20.5	18.8	19.7	18.1	19.8	18.8	20.2	21.5	20.1	20.9	17.5
1973	21.0	19.6	20.3	19.5	20.2	19.8	21.0	22.2	20.1	21.4	19.9
1972	21.3	21.6	21.4	20.8	19.9	20.4	21.8	20.6	24.6	22.2	20.5
1971	22.5	20.6	21.6	21.3	21.8	21.5	21.0	20.8	21.9	21.2	19.3
1970	21.9	20.9	21.4	20.4	21.3	20.8	20.9	20.1	23.1	21.2	19.0
1969	20.7	22.0	21.3	21.1	20.2	20.7	22.3	21.7	22.9	22.1	20.7
1968	22.1	21.4	21.5	19.6	19.6	19.0	21.4	21.2	21.4	21.3	22.1
1967	22.6	22.1	22.4	19.4	20.3	19.8	21.6	20.3	22.2	21.0	22.7
1966	23.0	22.8	22.7	21.6	21.5	20.8	24.6	23.9	25.0	24.8	23.8
1965	24.7	22.8	23.7	22.3	21.6	21.2	24.6	24.7	24.7	24.7	24.2
1964	23.4	21.7	22.7	22.1	22.1	22.1	24.5	23.3	25.2	23.9	25.3
1963	24.6	22.4	23.6	21.5	23.4	22.4	25.5	25.8	25.6	25.7	24.5
1962	24.0	23.3	23.7	21.9	22.6	22.2	27.3	26.7	29.0	27.5	26.7
1961	23.8	22.3	23.1	21.7	22.3	22.0	25.9	25.0	28.1	26.0	24.9
1960	23.6	23.8	23.7	21.4	25.0	23.0	27.3	27.1	28.7	27.9	26.0

"–" = Data not yet published or available.

Table 6 (continued)
Suicide Rates Among Elderly Age Groupings

MALES

YEAR	55–9	60–4	55–64	65–9	70–4	65–74	75+	75–9	80–4	75–84	85+
1980	24.9	23.9	24.4	28.1	33.5	30.2	43.5	41.5	43.8	42.0	50.6
1979	24.2	25.3	26.6	29.7	33.8	31.4	45.3	46.7	49.2	47.6	44.7
1978	25.4	30.1	27.5	30.2	37.2	33.1	47.7	45.9	50.6	47.6	48.3
1977	28.2	30.4	29.2	31.9	39.3	34.9	45.3	45.9	44.3	45.3	45.8
1976	29.4	30.3	29.8	32.3	36.4	34.0	43.6	41.6	44.5	42.7	47.5
1975	30.2	30.1	30.2	32.4	35.5	33.7	42.7	42.5	41.3	42.0	46.2
1974	30.7	29.7	30.2	30.5	36.4	32.9	43.8	42.5	45.2	43.5	45.2
1973	30.4	30.7	30.5	33.1	36.6	34.5	44.6	43.7	43.2	43.5	50.3
1972	30.2	33.1	31.5	35.3	36.7	35.9	45.9	39.6	54.2	45.0	50.0
1971	33.9	31.4	32.8	34.5	38.9	36.4	44.6	41.3	46.4	43.3	44.9
1970	32.8	32.5	32.7	34.8	37.5	36.0	43.2	39.3	49.1	42.8	42.4
1969	30.9	35.0	32.7	34.5	36.1	35.2	43.0	42.3	47.6	44.3	47.3
1968	33.3	34.0	33.6	33.4	33.8	33.6	44.7	41.2	46.4	43.0	54.1
1967	33.9	35.0	34.4	30.6	35.9	32.9	46.4	38.5	46.3	41.3	50.9
1966	34.4	38.0	36.0	34.9	36.5	35.6	51.0	47.4	54.0	49.7	58.2
1965	36.4	38.1	37.1	35.5	37.5	36.2	49.2	47.0	50.6	48.2	54.5
1964	35.5	36.7	36.1	34.7	37.6	37.0	50.5	46.1	53.6	47.5	59.3
1963	37.6	36.8	37.3	34.6	41.0	38.3	51.3	49.0	52.9	49.3	55.8
1962	37.8	38.2	38.0	36.9	40.0	38.2	54.8	51.6	59.4	54.2	58.3
1961	38.3	36.5	37.5	36.0	39.4	37.4	51.7	47.5	57.3	50.7	56.8
1960	37.5	38.5	38.0	36.4	43.7	39.5	52.7	49.3	57.4	52.0	56.8

FEMALES

YEAR	55–9	60–4	55–64	65–9	70–4	65–74	75+	75–9	80–4	75–84	85+
1980	8.6	8.2	8.4	6.6	6.4	6.5	5.4	5.9	4.7	5.4	5.5
1979	9.7	9.6	9.6	7.9	6.8	7.4	6.1	7.8	6.1	7.1	4.5
1978	10.8	8.4	9.7	8.3	7.4	7.9	6.8	9.0	6.0	7.4	5.1
1977	11.2	9.7	10.5	9.0	8.3	8.7	6.4	7.5	6.8	7.2	4.2
1976	12.3	9.9	11.1	8.6	8.2	8.4	6.9	7.6	7.0	7.4	5.4
1975	11.9	10.0	11.0	8.9	8.9	8.9	6.7	7.5	7.3	7.4	4.4
1974	11.2	9.3	10.3	8.3	7.6	8.0	6.2	7.7	5.7	6.9	3.8
1973	12.4	9.9	11.2	8.6	8.2	8.5	6.8	8.0	6.6	7.4	4.6
1972	13.1	11.6	12.4	9.2	7.7	8.5	7.1	7.9	7.1	7.6	5.4
1971	12.2	11.2	11.7	10.4	9.2	9.9	6.4	7.2	6.5	7.0	3.8
1970	12.0	10.7	11.4	8.8	9.2	9.0	6.7	7.0	6.9	7.0	5.9
1969	11.3	10.6	11.0	9.9	8.4	9.2	6.7	7.4	6.7	7.1	4.4
1968	11.3	9.9	10.6	7.6	7.2	7.5	6.1	7.1	5.3	6.5	4.5
1967	12.3	10.6	11.5	10.1	8.5	9.4	6.5	7.1	5.8	6.6	5.5
1966	11.0	10.2	10.6	9.2	8.6	8.9	6.6	7.7	6.5	7.2	4.0
1965	11.9	10.5	11.3	10.0	8.0	9.1	7.5	8.0	7.2	7.7	6.6
1964	10.7	9.6	10.2	10.0	8.8	9.8	6.1	6.8	6.0	6.4	4.1
1963	11.1	10.5	10.9	9.3	8.4	9.1	7.0	7.9	6.6	7.4	5.0
1962	10.3	10.5	10.4	8.2	7.9	8.2	7.3	7.1	7.5	7.2	7.3
1961	9.8	9.7	9.7	8.9	7.9	8.5	6.8	7.2	7.3	7.2	4.9
1960	10.1	10.2	10.2	8.0	8.8	8.4	8.2	9.2	7.9	8.9	6.0

Figure 1
Contribution of the Elderly to U.S. Suicide and Population, 1900–1983

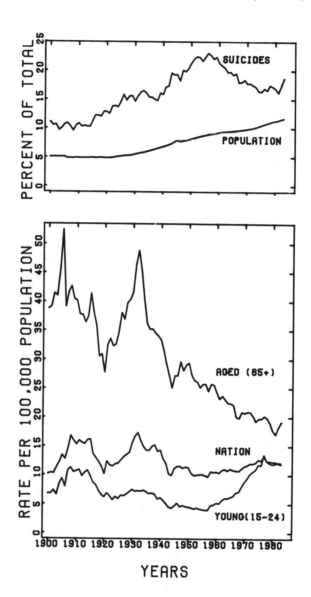

Figure 2
Elderly (65+) Suicide in the U.S. by Sex, 1933–1978

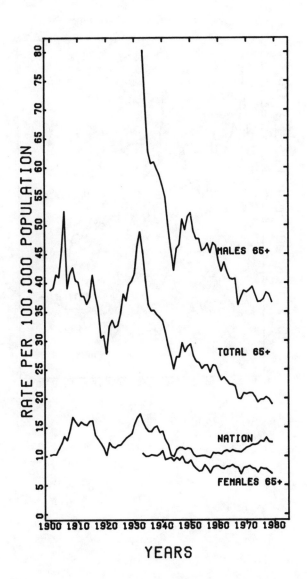

YEARS

Figure 3
Elderly (65+) Suicide in the U.S. by Race, 1933–1978

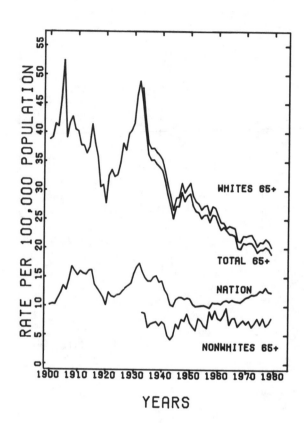

Figure 4
Suicide Among the Young-Old and Old-Old by Sex and Race, 1933–1978

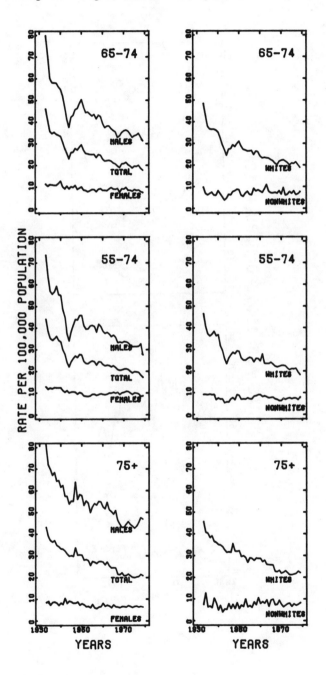

Figure 5
Suicide Among Old–Old Age Groups by Sex, 1933–1978

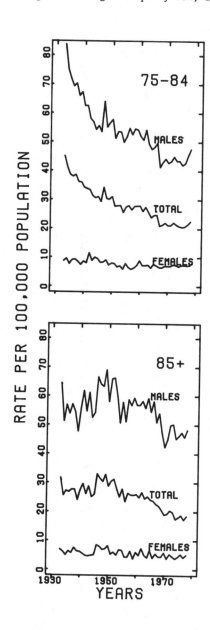

AUTHOR INDEX

The following index entries include names of authors and individuals appearing in reference citations as well as in text and annotations. Entries for which a single digit (2 through 5) is followed by a dash ("-") and then three digits refer to the number of the annotated references appearing in Chapters 2 through 5 and numbered consecutively from 001 within each chapter. Similarly, references in the demographic appendix are preceded by the letter "A" and a dash. Numbers that are not predeced by a single digit or letter and a dash refer to page numbers in the book.

Abel, Ernest L., 4-001
Abrahams, Ruby R., 13, 117, 3-037, 4-002
Achte, Kalle, 4-052
Acuff, F. Gene, 3-031
Adelson, Lester, 4-025
Ahlburg, Dennis A., 25, 4-003
Akiskai, H. S., 14, 30
Albala, A. A., 30
Altergott, K., 26, 27, 28
Alvarez, W. C., 21, 28
American Association of Retired Persons, 18, 28
American Association of Suicidology, 20
Anderson, S., 30
Anderson, William F., 4-022
Andress, V. R., 3, 28
Anger, H., 5-001
Aronson, Miriam K., 31, 47
Atchley, Robert C., 7, 17, 26, 28, 4-004
Atkinson, Maxwell, 4, 100, 166, 4-005
Aubry, H., 5-002

Bahn, Anita, K., 10, 4-026

Bahwens, E. E., 30
Bagley, Christopher, 87, 97, 4-006, 4-007
Baker, Frank, 13, 3-037
Balance, William D. G., 115, 4-043
Baldeschi, A., 5-067
Barakat, Samia, 4-013
Barraclough, B. M., 166, 3-001, 4-090
Barrett, C. J., 19, 28
Barrington, M. R., 22, 28
Basson, M. D., 20, 28
Bassuk, E. L., 75
Batchelor, I. R. C., 12, 41, 122, 123, 3-002, 3-003, 4-008
Battin, Margaret P., 20, 23, 28, 29, 32, 33, 34, 35
Baum, P., 5-037
Beck, Aaron T., 14, 29, 4-048
Beckwith, B. P., 21, 29
Bennett, A. E., 13, 15, 3-004
Bennett, Ruth, 31, 47
Benson, Roger A., 3-005
Berardo, F. M., 10, 29
Berdes, Celia, 15, 26, 3-006
Berezin, Martin A., 30, 3-019
Berg, Robert C., 98

SUBJECT INDEX

The numbers appearing in this index refer to the page on which the topic was mentioned. Some topics were mentioned in almost every work on elderly suicide, for example, depression, loneliness, etc. For that reason, only citations for which there was major coverage or emphasis on topics are listed for many terms.

About the Compilers

NANCY J. OSGOOD is Assistant Professor of Gerontology and Sociology at the Medical College of Virginia, Richmond. She is the author of *Seniors on Stage: The Impact of Creative Dramatics on the Elderly, Aging: Issues and Policies for the '80s*, and *Elderly Suicide: A Practitioner's Guide to Diagnosis and Intervention*. Her articles have been published in *Geriatric Medicine Today, Society and Leisure*, the *Journal of Minority Aging*, and the *Journal of Applied Gerontology*.

JOHN L. MCINTOSH is Associate Professor of Psychology at Indiana University at South Bend and a Research Associate at the Center for Gerontological Education, Research, and Services, University of Notre Dame. He is the author of *Research on Suicide: A Bibliography* (Greenwood Press, 1985) and the compiler of several extensive bibliographies on various aspects of suicide. He has contributed articles to *Suicide: Assessment and Intervention, Omega, Suicide and Life-Threatening Behavior, Journal of Gerontological Social Work*, and the *International Journal of Aging and Human Development*.